ADVANCES IN
Vascular Surgery®

VOLUME 11

ADVANCES IN
Vascular Surgery®

VOLUMES 1 THROUGH 9 (OUT OF PRINT)

VOLUME 10

ADVANCES IN

Vascular Surgery®

VOLUME 11

Editor-in-Chief
K. Craig Kent, MD, FACS
Professor of Surgery and Chief, Division of Vascular Surgery, New
York–Presbyterian Hospital, Weill Medical College of Cornell University,
Columbia University College of Physicians & Surgeons, New York,
New York

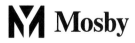 Mosby

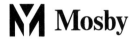 Mosby

Vice President, Continuity Publishing: Timothy M. Griswold
Managing Editor: David Orzechowski
Developmental Editor: Beth Martz
Senior Manager, Continuity Production: Idelle L. Winer
Issue Manager: Donna Skelton

Printed in the United States of America
Composition by Thomas Technology Solutions, Inc.
Printing/binding by Sheridan Books, Inc.

Editorial Office:
Elsevier
300 East
170 South Independence Mall West
Philadelphia, PA 19106-3399

International Standard Serial Number: 1069-7292
International Standard Book Number: 0-323-02099-2

Contributors

Michael T. Caps, MD, MPH
Division of Vascular Therapy, Hawaii Permanente Medical Group, Honolulu, Hawaii

Daniel G. Clair, MD
Vice Chairman, Department of Vascular Surgery, The Cleveland Clinic Foundation, Cleveland, Ohio

Rajeev Dayal, MD
Fellow in Vascular Surgery, Department of Surgery, Division of Vascular Surgery, The New York-Presbyterian Hospital, Weill Medical College of Cornell University, New York, New York

Peter L. Faries, MD, FACS
Chief of Endovascular Surgery, Division of Vascular Surgery, New York-Presbyterian Hospital, Cornell University, Weill Medical College, Columbia University, College of Physicians and Surgeons, New York, New York

Michael A. Golden, MD
Associate Professor of Surgery, University of Pennsylvania School of Medicine, Chief, Vascular Surgery, University of Pennsylvania Medical Center–Presbyterian, Philadelphia, Pennsylvania

Richard M. Green, MD
Professor of Surgery, Lenox Hill Hospital, New York, New York

Neal C. Hadro
New York-Presbyterian Hospital, New York, New York

Peter Henderson, BA
Vascular Research Fellow, Division of Vascular Surgery, New York–Presbyterian Hospital, Weill Medical College of Cornell University, Columbia University College of Physicians & Surgeons, New York, New York

K. Kasirajan, MD
Assistant Professor of Surgery, Department of Surgery, Emory University School of Medicine, Atlanta, Georgia

K. Craig Kent, MD, FACS
Professor of Surgery and Chief, Division of Vascular Surgery, New York–Presbyterian Hospital, Weill Medical College of Cornell University, Columbia University College of Physicians & Surgeons, New York, New York

John C. Lantis II, MD
Assistant Professor of Surgery, Columbia University College of Physicians and Surgeons, Assistant Attending in Surgery, New York Presbyterian Hospital, New York, New York

Nicholas J. Morrissey, MD
Assistant Professor of Surgery, Columbia/Weill Cornell Division of Vascular Surgery, New York, New York

Albeir Y. Mousa, MD
Vascular Research Fellow, Division of Vascular Surgery, New York–Presbyterian Hospital, Weill Medical College of Cornell University, Columbia University College of Physicians & Surgeons, New York, New York

Nicolas Nelken, MD
Division of Vascular Therapy, Hawaii Permanente Medical Group, Honolulu, Hawaii

Kenneth Ouriel, MD
Chairman, Department of Vascular Surgery, The Cleveland Clinic Foundation, Cleveland, Ohio

Peter A. Schneider, MD
Division of Vascular Therapy, Hawaii Permanente Medical Group, Honolulu, Hawaii

Michael B. Silva, Jr, MD, FACS
Professor of Surgery and Radiology, Department of Surgery, Division of Vascular Surgery and Vascular Interventional Radiology, Texas Tech University Health Sciences Center, Lubbock, Texas

Contents

CHAPTER 1

The Optimal Paradigm for Retraining Vascular Surgeons

Kenneth Ouriel, MD
Chairman, Department of Vascular Surgery, The Cleveland Clinic
Foundation, Cleveland, Ohio

Richard M. Green, MD
Professor of Surgery, Lenox Hill Hospital, New York, NY

ABSTRACT

Advances in the procedural oriented specialties such as surgery, interventional cardiology, and others are dependent on technologic innovation. As examples, coronary artery bypass surgery awaited the development of cardio-
pulmonary bypass machines, interventional cardiology blossomed after the
introduction of small-caliber balloons and stents, and endovascular aneurysm
repair became a reality after the mating of metallic stents with fabric grafts
and their delivery systems. After appropriate investigative analysis, technologic innovations must be introduced to the grassroots of the procedural specialties that care for patients with the disease groups, and can be addressed
with this technology. Introduction of new technology must proceed along 2
separate pathways. First, the attending physicians who teach residents and
fellows in training programs must become skilled at the procedures so that
these skills are transferred to new physicians entering the field. Second, the
skills must be taught to postgraduate physicians who have completed residency and fellowship training, but who have decades ahead of them with
which to use these techniques. The development of a vascular endosurgical
workforce will require a detailed analysis of the problem, identification of
endovascular surgeons with teaching interests and skills, creation of a sufficient number of suitable training sites, and a continuous evaluation of these
sites. The aim of this monograph is to describe a variety of options for the
training of endovascular surgeons. A scant amount of objective information is

available on which to base the design of such programs. For this reason, the information contained herein represents anecdotal experience from the initial attempts at endovascular training. In this regard, the "optimal" paradigm for retraining of vascular surgeons has yet to be defined and remains a topic of spirited debate.

The goal of modern health technology is to improve on existing methods of prevention, diagnosis, and treatment. Most technologic innovations represent small changes over existing practice and approach to clinical problems. In these cases, it is relatively easy for practitioners to adopt these relatively minor incremental changes to continue to keep up with the standards of care. In the case of vascular surgery, examples of such incremental changes that were relatively easy for the practitioners to implement included the use of Doppler ultrasound for the objective documentation of the severity of lower extremity occlusive disease, in situ techniques for lower extremity arterial reconstruction, and placement of a patch for arterial closure at the time of carotid endarterectomy. A cursory review of such examples reveals that after a comprehensive residency or fellowship program, vascular surgeons could easily keep up with changes in the field merely by reading a few articles or attending a few short courses.

The advent of endovascular procedures drastically changed the manner in which vascular disease could be treated. Endovascular treatments represented "disruptive technologies"; novel technologies that bring about drastic change in the manner in which we do things.[1] Clayton Christensen initially defined disruptive technologies as "simple, and convenient to use innovations that are initially used only by the unsophisticated," but the term has come to mean a competitive technology that rapidly transforms the marketplace. As such, percutaneous endovascular therapies are clearly "disruptive"; they hold the potential to replace many of the traditional open surgical procedures that vascular surgeons and their patients have become accustomed to. If the vascular surgical community does not embrace these new technologies, other specialties will. To continue to care for the patient with vascular disease, vascular surgeons must attain proficiency in the use of endovascular technologies.

In distinction to previous innovations from the 1960s, 70s, and 80s, practicing vascular surgeons are often ill-equipped to perform new endovascular techniques that appeared over the last decade.[2] Unlike novel open surgical techniques, the training of contemporary vascular surgeons never included the guidewire and catheter skills necessary to be an accomplished endovascular practitioner. In fact, much of the equipment and techniques never existed at the time most vascular surgeons were in training. Also, the modalities are sufficiently complex to require dedicated endovascular training to attain proficiency. No longer can vascular surgeons merely read an article or attend a course to become proficient in the new technique; a dedicated period of hands-on training is necessary.

TRAINING PARADIGMS

How can vascular surgeons acquire the necessary skills to provide state-of-the-art endovascular options for their patients? There exist 3 potential paradigms for "retraining": self-teaching, ad hoc training, and a dedicated training program. In actuality, these activities comprise "primary training" rather than "retraining paradigms," since many of the techniques and procedures are new to most vascular surgeons and were never part of their fellowship training programs.[2,3]

SELF-TEACHING

Much of what we do as vascular surgeons is "self-taught." This is especially true for innovators who develop new techniques not yet in widespread acceptance. This mode of training has been the tradition since the beginnings of our specialty, and it works well for those procedures that are relatively close in scope to accepted procedures. For example, vascular surgeons skilled in the performance of carotid endarterectomy with primary closure of the arteriotomy had no problem in adapting the procedure to patch closure. The procedure of carotid endarterectomy was no different, and surgeons were already skilled in the patch closure of other noncarotid arteries. To use the techniques of patch closure at a new location, the carotid endarterectomy site, was easy, straightforward, and something that could be self-taught. Endovascular procedures, by contrast, encompass a field sufficiently distinct from the traditional open surgical procedures such that self-teaching is usually inefficient. The self-taught trainee usually experiences problems, both with respect to patient selection and technical skills that had been previously elucidated through the experience of others. To incorporate an overused idiom, the trainee "relearns the wheel."

AD HOC TRAINING

Practitioners fortunate enough to be part of a group with at least one person skilled in endovascular techniques may be able to train additional group members on an "ad hoc" basis. In most cases, the unskilled members of the group scrub with the training member, much like a fellowship program. In some cases, the trainee may choose to work with other specialists who are skilled in endovascular techniques. For instance, the trainee may choose to spend time in interventional radiology or cardiology. Such a paradigm may work well in particular situations, but this pathway is far from ideal.[4,5] Experience has demonstrated that surgeons are best trained by surgeons. That said, this particular pathway may be best for certain new techniques, for instance, carotid stenting. The technique of carotid stenting requires the use of 0.014-in systems, a platform unfamiliar to most vascular surgeons. Moreover, aspects of the technique are similar to those used for coronary interventions, specifically with respect to the use of guiding catheters and monorail systems. Noting the paucity of vascular surgeons proficient in such techniques, the initial training might be most efficiently accomplished by an interventional cardiologist. Once enough vascular surgeons have been trained in these techniques, the training can then be performed by these individuals.

In general, an ad hoc training paradigm is much less efficient than one in which the trainee dedicates a continuous period of training toward endovascular procedures. Ad hoc training paradigms may place days or weeks between endovascular cases, allowing time to forget what was learned. It is intuitive that frequent repetition of a given task provides the most efficient means for learning. For this reason, it is advantageous to dedicate a continuous period toward endovascular training.

DEDICATED TRAINING PROGRAM

The most efficient means of learning endovascular techniques is to dedicate a specified period to "train." Of course, it is usually difficult to set aside one's vascular surgical practice to devote the time necessary for training. Such a paradigm has been easiest to accomplish for group practitioners, where the other group members are willing to cover for the training individual.

Several programs throughout the United States have organized training programs where interested persons can enroll in a dedicated program of endovascular training.[6] Some of these programs have focused on practicing vascular surgeons, whereas others enroll vascular fellows who cannot obtain adequate training at their home institution. It is imperative that these adjunctive fellowships or "minifellowships" do not compete with the training of the institution's formal vascular fellowship program approved by the Accreditation Council for Graduate Medical Education (ACGME). Thus, each institution should have ample volume to provide sufficient case volumes for the ACGME-approved fellows as well as the adjunctive endovascular trainees.

Part and parcel of training is an evaluation and certification process to ensure that the program will provide the trainee with an adequate educational experience. The Society of Vascular Surgery organized a committee to certify endovascular training programs, the Endovascular Program Evaluation and Endorsement Committee (EV-PEEC).[7] Centers apply to EV-PEEC and a site visit is conducted. After a review that includes observation of endovascular cases, the center can be endorsed as a comprehensive site for endovascular training. Although the EV-PEEC bylaws state that the organization shall serve as the body that confers endorsement on institutions offering endovascular training to vascular surgeons either as a component of an ACGME-accredited training program or as a free-standing postfellowship experience, the program has thus far been applied only to adjunctive postfellowship programs.

Several questions arise with respect to the specifics of the dedicated training program. First, what should the duration of training be to gain adequate experience? Second, where should the training be performed? Third, who should perform the training? And lastly, is a contiguous period of time necessary, or can the training program be split into discontinuous segments? The remainder of this chapter is dedicated to a discussion of these questions.

DURATION OF TRAINING

The optimal duration for endovascular training is dependent on a multiplicity of parameters, including the prior experience of the trainee in diagnostic and interventional techniques, the manual dexterity of the individual, the amount of independent experience given to the trainee, the number of other trainees competing for a limited pool of clinical material, and the number and complexity of cases the trainee is exposed to during the training period. An ideal training site would provide the trainee with exposure to endovascular cases of graded complexity, beginning with basic techniques and progressing to complex diagnostic cannulations, and lastly, interventional techniques. In most settings, however, such a graded experience is not feasible. Case scheduling can never be planned on the basis of complexity; straightforward cases will be interspersed with technically challenging cases. Nevertheless, trainees can be given more independence with the less challenging cases early on, with increasing independence given as their skills advance.

The ACGME designated endovascular procedures as an important component of vascular surgical training, and the Vascular Surgery Board of the American Board of Surgery (VSB-ABS) has been delegated as the responsible entity for all board-related vascular training issues pertaining to ACGME-approved residencies and fellowships.[8] A full year of dedicated endovascular training would likely provide most individuals with competency in a broad array of endovascular techniques. Whereas a 1-year duration may be feasible within a formal vascular surgical fellowship, this paradigm is impractical for most practicing vascular surgeons. Instead, shorter training programs have been organized to balance the impracticality of longer programs with the educational inadequacy of shorter paradigms. At present, a 3-month period of dedicated training appears to offer an acceptable arrangement that will achieve these goals.[2]

TRAINING CURRICULA

Any training curriculum must begin with a review of the pathophysiology of the diseases, the indications for intervention, and the expectations for clinical outcome. Technical skills should be taught only after the trainee has acquired a broad fund of knowledge about the disease. Fortunately, most practicing vascular surgeons already possess this clinical knowledge at the time they begin an endovascular training program.

Next, the trainee should develop skill in the interpretation of diagnostic imaging studies, to include ultrasound, computed tomography (CT) and magnetic resonance imaging (MRI), and traditional angiography. The trainee should become familiar with normal anatomy as well as the abnormal variants. The trainee should know when to use lateral views, craniocaudal orientation, and right or left obliquities to afford the best imaging of a particular vascular segment. Lastly, the trainee must spend a great deal of time dedicated to the development of a comprehensive portfolio of endovascular technical skills. These skills run the gamut from vascular access through stenting and deployment of embolic protection devices (Table 1).

No amount of textbook studying or classroom-based didactic lectures can hone the technical skills that comprise endovascular procedures. Initially, animal and cadaver models were created to provide a setting where the trainee might begin to develop these skills without risk to the patient. Many of these in vivo models offered realistic analogues to the clinical setting, but the training was often expensive and always inefficient. Animal and cadaver models provide a limited number of vascular segments available for intervention, and each intervention consumed expensive catheters, wires, balloons, and stents. Moreover, fluoroscopic imaging equipment and contrast was necessary, further increasing the cost of training and exposing the trainee to radiation, albeit mild.

More recently, computerized simulators have been developed to aid the trainee in acquiring technical skills. Such systems provide hands-on teaching, using computerized libraries of modules based on real patient information and precise representations of the mechanical properties of specific catheters and wires. There exist 2 general aspects of simulators, each of which has been addressed to a varying extent by the different simulator manufacturers: (1) the de-

TABLE 1.
Spectrum of Procedures That Should Be Included in a Comprehensive
Endovascular Training Program*

Gaining vascular access
　　　　Basic cannulation of access vessels (femoral, brachial)
　　　　Micropuncture techniques, including ultrasound-guided access
Basic angiographic techniques
　　　　Injection rates, filming rates, obliquities
　　　　Radiation safety
Placement of sheaths
　　　　Short sheath placement
　　　　Sheaths that go over the aortic bifurcation
　　　　Long sheaths, shaped sheaths, and guide catheters
　　　　Touhy-Borst valves
Wires
　　　　Use of standard 0.035 and 0.014 guidewires
　　　　Hydrophilic wires
　　　　Snares
Balloons
　　　　Standard over the wire balloons
　　　　Rapid exchange (monorail) balloons
Stents (bare and covered)
　　　　Balloon-expandable
　　　　Self-expanding
Emboli protection devices
Aortic stent grafts
Thrombus management
　　　　Thrombolytic catheters and infusion wires
　　　　Mechanical thrombectomy devices
Embolization procedures (hypogastric, endoleaks, direct sac puncture)
　　　　Coils
　　　　Glue

* The list is not comprehensive.

gree to which the simulator's appearance replicates a true angiography suite, and (2) the degree to which the product simulates the visual and tactile properties of the angiographic procedure. The former property attains greatest importance when training angiographic technologists and nurses. For such persons, the appearance of the suite is of greater importance than the tactile properties of the procedure. For such trainees, an authentic depiction of the angiography suite is the overriding goal. By contrast, the appearance of the suite is less relevant when training endovascular surgeons. Rather, a true representation of the tactile properties of the catheters, the wires, and their interactions with the vascular anatomy is of paramount importance.

Simulators provide the opportunity to perform large numbers of procedures without risk to patients. No simulator can provide an absolutely precise representation of an actual clinical procedure, but the newer machines provide a mechanism for practicing endovascular techniques to develop the necessary technical skills in a rapid, efficient, and cost-effective manner. With software improvements and the creation of large libraries of clinical cases, it is likely that simulator technology will play an increasingly important role in the training of endovascular specialists. The learning can occur at times determined by the trainee and can be semi-independent.

CREDENTIALING

Although credentialing activities are always local (hospital-determined), training paradigms must take societal recommendations into account.[9] As well, the process for admission into training programs should consider applicant-specific issues of credentialing. At a time when the demand for training outstrips supply, enrollment of individuals who will have great difficulty in obtaining privileges for endovascular techniques impedes the objective to expand the endovascular workforce. Successful applicants to training programs should also demonstrate a high probability of being granted access to appropriate angiographic equipment at their home institution.

There exists a variety of credentialing guideline documents, each specific to a particular society whose members are engaged in endovascular procedures.[10,11] The most recent document, prepared by an ad hoc committee of the American Association for Vascular Surgery and the Society for Vascular Surgery (SVS), defines precisely what vascular surgery is, and outlines the scope of vascular surgical activities that should be addressed by any training program.[8] This article makes reference to a previous SVS document from 1999 that included a minimal requirement of 50 angiograms

TABLE 2.
Credentialing Guidelines for Interventional Procedures, as Published by the Radiology, Cardiology, and Vascular Surgery Societies

	SCVIR	SCAI	ACC*	AHA*	SVS/ISCVS* (1993)	SVS/ISCVS* (1998)
Catheterizations /angiograms	200	100/50†	100	100	50†	100/50†
Interventions	25	50/25†	50/25†	50/25†	10 to 15†	50/25†
Live demonstration	yes	yes	yes	yes	yes	yes

* Includes knowledge of thrombolysis or thrombolytic therapy.
† As primary interventionist.
Abbreviations: *SCVIR*, Society of Cardiovascular and Interventional Radiology; *SCAI*, Society for Cardiac Angiography and Interventions; *ACC*, American College of Cardiology; *AHA*, American Heart Association; *SVS/ISCVS*, Society for Vascular Surgery/International Society for Cardiovascular Surgery.
(Courtesy of White RA, Hodgson KJ, Ahn SS, et al: Endovascular interventions training and credentialing for vascular surgeons. *J Vasc Surg* 29:177-186, 1999. Reprinted with permission.)

and 25 interventions with the surgeon as the primary interventionalist (Table 2).[3] The authors note that a mentored experience should be obtained before independence, and the aforementioned minimal numerical requirements do not include these cases.

LEGAL IMPLICATIONS

There exist legal implications related to training programs. Legal hurdles must be crossed to protect the trainee, the trainer, and the training institution. These legal implications are usually state-specific, but some general guidelines apply to most locales. In all instances, legal counsel should be obtained before the organization of a training program.

Whenever a hands-on training is planned, the trainee should have some form of liability coverage. The easiest manner in which to arrange such malpractice coverage is to place the individual on the institution's coverage policy for its residents. This is not always possible, and in many centers trainees must arrange for their own coverage. In some cases, the trainee's current malpractice policy will cover liability at the training site. It is safest to notify the carrier of the trainee's plans in writing if such an arrangement is contemplated. Of importance, in no case should the trainee be allowed to perform completely independent procedures without the training physician in attendance. In most cases, the amount of independence should be somewhat less than that provided to standard vascular fellows.

Even when a hands-on clinical experience is not a part of the program, legal issues related to the Health Insurance Portability and Accountability Act (HIPAA) guidelines are existent. Patient confidentiality is important, and it may be reasonable to have the training individuals complete the institution's HIPAA training before beginning the program. If the trainee is part of investigational protocols, it is also important for that individual to complete the institution's clinical trial training modules. Many of these programs are web-based and can be completed before or just after arriving at the training institution.

SUMMARY

Novel innovations are being introduced into the practice of endovascular surgery at an increasing rate. These innovations drastically decrease the invasiveness of vascular therapies, sometimes at the cost of long-term durability. Patients and their physicians are willing, however, to accept a slight decrement in long-term outcome to avoid a major open surgical procedure. Also, the durability of endovascular techniques will improve over time. Thus, if vascular surgeons are to continue to participate in the care of patients with vascular disease, they must become proficient in these new therapeutic modalities.

Retraining of vascular surgeons is of paramount importance in this goal. Although a variety of training paradigms exist, a few common principles apply. First, the acquisition of endovascular skills is accelerated if the trainee can devote a dedicated period to the program. Second, such training is best accomplished by skilled endovascular surgeons, rather than relegating training to nonsurgical specialists who have primary educational responsibilities for residents and fellows in their own specialty. Third, the trainee should seek to become proficient in the interpretation of imaging studies such as MR, CT, and angiography, as such proficiency is necessary for the planning of endovascular interventions and to gauge success or failure over long-term follow-up. Lastly, trainees should focus very early on the granting of endovascular privileges at their home institution, with access to equipment adequate to perform the myriad procedures that encompass the practice of endovascular surgery.

Once an adequate workforce of endovascular surgeons has been developed, the major thrust of training will again be transferred to the standard vascular surgical fellowship programs. With an adequate foundation in endovascular techniques at the grassroots level, new techniques can be assimilated in less formal fashion. Once our educational goals have been achieved, the incorporation of new endovascular techniques can revert to methods similar to those that we use to integrate new open surgical techniques, with greater emphasis on self-teaching and independent learning. This observation will be the litmus test for whether the specialty of vascular surgery has achieved its goal of training an adequate number of "endo-competent" surgeons.

REFERENCES

1. Christensen CM, Bohmer R, Kenagy B, et al: Will disruptive innovations cure health care? *Harv Business Rev* September-October:102-111, 2000.
2. Ouriel K, Kent KC: The role of the vascular surgeon in endovascular procedures. *J Vasc Surg* 33:902-903, 2001.
3. White RA, Hodgson KJ, Ahn SS, et al: Endovascular interventions training and credentialing for vascular surgeons. *J Vasc Surg* 29:177-186, 1999.
4. Green RM: Collaboration between vascular surgeons and interventional radiologists: Reflections after two years. *J Vasc Surg* 31:826-830, 2000.
5. Green RM: A time for co-opetition. *J Vasc Surg* 28:955-963, 1998.
6. Wieslander CK, Huang CC, Omura MC, et al: Endovascular workforce for peripheral vascular disease: Current and future needs. *J Vasc Surg* 35:1218-1225, 2002.
7. Endovascular PEEC bylaws, http://www.vascularweb.org/file/EV-EEC _31-36.pdf, 2003. Endovascular Committee, Society for Vascular Surgery-Accessed July 5, 2004.
8. Moore WS, Clagett GP, Veith FJ, et al: Guidelines for hospital privileges in vascular surgery: An update by an ad hoc committee of the American Association for Vascular Surgery and the Society for Vascular Surgery. *J Vasc Surg* 36:1276-1282, 2002.
9. LoGerfo FW: A "four plus" future for general surgery and vascular surgery: Maintaining the union. *J Vasc Surg* 35:1073-1077, 2002.
10. White RA, Hodgson KJ, Ahn SS, et al: Endovascular interventions training and credentialing for vascular surgeons. *J Vasc Surg* 29:177-186, 1999.
11. White RA, Fogarty TJ, Baker WH, et al: Endovascular surgery credentialing and training for vascular surgeons. *J Vasc Surg* 17:1095-1102, 1993.

C HAPTER 2

How to Start and Build an Endovascular Program

Peter A. Schneider, MD
Division of Vascular Therapy, Hawaii Permanente Medical Group, Honolulu

Michael T. Caps, MD, MPH
Division of Vascular Therapy, Hawaii Permanente Medical Group, Honolulu

Nicolas Nelken, MD
Division of Vascular Therapy, Hawaii Permanente Medical Group, Honolulu

S tarting an endovascular program is a first step. The real goal is to integrate endovascular techniques and concepts into vascular practice. In the not too distant future, the concept of vascular "surgery" is not likely to be functional. The most effective vascular specialists will be those who provide a full spectrum of management options including prevention, medical management, endovascular therapy, and open surgery. Even now, the concept of a separate program for endovascular surgery is antithetical to the seamless care of patients for which we strive. Vascular disease management is gradually approaching a stage in which endovascular surgery will be the treatment of choice for most situations requiring mechanical intervention, with open surgery reserved for endovascular failures and those patients with the absolute worst disease morphology. Endovascular techniques have dramatically influenced the care of disease in every vascular bed. As the sophistication of these techniques advances, the maturation of the field of endovascular surgery does likewise. The opportunity to relieve suffering, reduce morbidity, and manage threatening illness with less invasive approaches is truly a privilege.

WHY START AN ENDOVASCULAR PROGRAM?

The short answer to the above question is: most vascular disease will probably be treated this way, and it's usually to the patients' benefit.

In the prestent era, endovascular intervention was more of a curiosity than an integral treatment modality for noncoronary vascular disease. The results of treatment were best in patients who needed these procedures least. The most appropriate lesions were focal, nonorificial stenoses of the common iliac artery, superficial femoral artery, or renal artery. Nevertheless, there was a high rate of immediate failure because of residual stenosis and dissection, and a nonnegligible rate of patients requiring emergency surgery for organ or lower extremity ischemia. Orifice lesions, complex stenoses, occlusions, and embolizing lesions were not well treated with balloon angioplasty alone, and attempting one of these sometimes led to worsening ischemia. Carotid, visceral, diffuse femoral-popliteal, and most renal and tibial occlusive disease and aneurysms could not be satisfactorily treated in the prestent era without open surgery.

With the development of stents has come the ability to extend endovascular solutions to treat many of these lesions without a significant incidence of immediate failure, emergency open repair, or a worsening of the clinical condition. The development of stents has led to the further development of stent-grafts, and in the near future, drug-eluting stents will likely reach clinical utility. Endovascular surgery has matured substantially over the past decade and is now the primary mode of therapy for many disease presentations, including renal artery stenosis, aortoiliac occlusive disease, many patients with infrainguinal occlusive disease, and aortic aneurysms. The only major vascular bed where endovascular intervention has not played a prominent role in the past decade is the extracranial cerebrovascular circulation. As the results of carotid stent trials become available, it is likely that endovascular surgery will assume an increasing role in the treatment of carotid bifurcation stenosis.[1]

Numerous factors have promoted the development and maturation of the field of endovascular surgery. The most important of these factors are discussed below.

1.   A dramatic change in attitude has occurred among vascular specialists over the past 10 years about the utility and potential long-term benefit of endovascular techniques.[2-6]
2.   Endovascular skills have rapidly improved among vascular specialists, providing a conduit for new approaches among practitioners who may have in the past, only provided the option of traditional surgery. Vascular surgeons have also recognized the

importance of maintaining an endovascular inventory and also the need for proper imaging equipment.

3. There has been continuous improvement in technology and in the tools available for the treatment of vascular disease through endoluminal manipulation. This improved technology is manifested in the form of:

    a. Better imaging with both stationary and portable systems
    b. Improved guidewires and catheters, including small platform and monorail systems
    c. Better stent technology including balloon-expandable, self-expanding covered stents, low-profile stents, and soon, drug-eluting stents
    d. Alternative methods of recanalization, such as thrombolysis, subinitimal angioplasty, and hydrophilic guidewires and catheters
    e. Better devices for access including guiding sheaths and closure devices

4. Preoperative imaging techniques including duplex mapping and magnetic resonance arteriography help to select patients for endovascular therapy before the performance of arteriography.[7,8]

5. There is a substantial increase in awareness of minimally invasive surgery and its benefits across all surgical specialties. Patients, primary physicians, and specialists in other nonvascular disciplines have come to expect the development and the benefits of this dramatic transition to less invasive intervention.

PLANNING, INITIATING, AND GROWING AN ENDOVASCULAR PROGRAM

In this section, we review the various factors that must be included in planning, initiating, and growing an endovascular program. These factors are:

- Developing endovascular skills
- Obtaining hospital privileges to perform endovascular procedures
- Planning for and obtaining imaging equipment
- Procuring and maintaining endovascular inventory
- Establishing the scope of practice
- Understanding the market for endovascular procedures
- Handling institutional politics
- Assessing outcomes
- Planning for the future

DEVELOPING ENDOVASCULAR SKILLS

Just a little over a decade ago, endovascular skills consisted mostly of the ability to pass a guidewire and catheter and perform an arteriogram or a balloon angioplasty of the iliac or superficial femoral artery. Many special procedures suites functioned based on cut film without the use of digital imaging. Access devices for endovascular therapy were primitive by today's standards, and stents were not available. Because of a dramatic increase in the available techniques, the skills to perform endovascular surgery have also reached a new level of complexity. Performing iliac artery balloon angioplasty is essential to endovascular practice, but it is only the beginning. There are now available many aids that are useful in helping to orient and train surgeons in endovascular skills.[9-11]

Obtaining endovascular skills is significantly different from obtaining hospital privileges; the latter is addressed in the next section. An important part of obtaining endovascular skills is the need to become familiar with the inventory and the various options available with respect to guidewires, catheters, access techniques, and methods of revascularization. Inventory is discussed in a section below.

The more developed the endovascular skills, the more likely the program will be successful. Endovascular skills may be homegrown or imported, and are now being taught in vascular fellowships.[2,12-14] The issue of training surgeons who are already in practice and do not have endovascular skills is a significant one and has been addressed by the Society for Vascular Surgery (SVS). Surgeons have used their enthusiasm and imagination to gain endovascular skills over the past few years, and there are many surgeons now who can teach these skills to others. The SVS has established a system of 3-month senior endovascular fellowships and an accreditation mechanism for these fellowships.

The arbitrary division of vascular reconstructions into endovascular and open has been a disservice to patients. A key pathway to obtaining endovascular skills is the potential use of fluoroscopic imaging, image-guided instrumentation, and endovascular techniques as an adjunct to open surgery. Many of the commonly performed open procedures can be improved by completion arteriography, fluoroscopy to guide catheter placement, or inflow or outflow balloon angioplasty. As these adjuncts become integrated into the treatment algorithms, they are likely to be used in more and different ways. Endovascular approaches include some skills, such as eye-fluoro-hand coordination, that may not seem intuitive. Although the learning curve for endovascular skills varies from one surgeon to

TABLE 1.
Minimum Case Requirements for Performing Endovascular Surgery

	SCVIR	SCAI	ACC	AHA	SVS/AAVS
Angiograms	200	100/50[a]	100	100	100/50*
Interventions	25	50/25[a]	50/25*	50/25*	50/25*

*As primary interventionist.
Abbreviations: SCVIR, Society of Cardiovascular and Interventional Radiology; *SCAI*, Society for Cardiac Angiography and Interventions; *ACC*, American College of Cardiology; *AHA*, American Heart Association; *SVS/AAVS*, Society for Vascular Surgery/American Association of Vascular Surgery. (Courtesy of Schneider PA: *Endovascular Skills*. New York, Marcel Dekker, Inc, 2003, p 4.)

another, surgeons are uniquely qualified to develop these skills because of familiarity with the anatomy, pathology, natural history of vascular disease, and the other treatment options.

No one knows the correct number of endovascular cases that is necessary to achieve competence. However, several societies, including the SVS, have issued minimum requirements (Table 1).[15-20] These numbers may be used to gain some perspective on how many cases are required to get started. Moreover, hospital credentialing committees sometimes use these numbers to establish requirements for hospital privileging. Basic skills are necessary to treat iliac and superficial femoral arteries and place vena cava filters. Complex aortic or tibial angioplasty requires a more developed skill set. Renal and carotid stenting are even more challenging since they involve remote access, short distance runoff (to anchor a guidewire), and unforgiving end organs. When you perform endovascular interventions as part of your practice, do not forget that you are competing with all other specialists who desire to perform endovascular interventions. In this setting, you must be able to show that your skills are excellent, that your results are satisfactory, and that your incorporation of new techniques and procedures is rational and well thought out.

Another challenge is to continue to improve and update one's skills after a certain minimum level of expertise has been attained. This maintenance of skills requires vigilance and enthusiasm, and includes maintaining inventory, continuing medical education, reading journals, taking notes at meetings, and having a network of colleagues with whom you can discuss a case or confer with when a difficult problem arises. As is the case with open surgery, endovascular procedures must be performed on a regular basis to allow maintenance of skills.

OBTAINING HOSPITAL PRIVILEGES TO PERFORM THE ENDOVASCULAR PROCEDURES

Hospital privileges are granted by each individual institution. Some institutions have specific criteria for endovascular procedures and others do not. Individual practitioners must check with their own institution to identify the specific requirements. Some institutions have set up committees that may be multidisciplinary in nature, that adjudicate endovascular privileging. If a multidisciplinary committee is set up, vascular surgeons should be represented, and although compromises are often appropriate, the emphasis should be on setting high standards.

When a contentious issue such as endovascular privileging arises, external standards, such as those published by various societies, are often used by hospital credentialing committees to define endovascular privileges (Table 1). Specific requirements for endovascular procedures should be specifically stated within the credentialing documents for your vascular department or the department of surgery at your institution, just as a set of criteria is established within your institution for granting privileges to perform carotid endarterectomy, lower extremity bypass, or other open vascular procedures. The standards in our department are summarized in Table 2. Regardless of how the endovascular privileges are established, the goal should be high, and as specialists in the field of vascular disease, we need to exceed that standard.

The more clearly and specifically these qualifications are stated, the better it is for vascular specialists. A problem in many institu-

TABLE 2.
Summary of Guidelines for Vascular Therapy Privileges at Kaiser Hospital Honolulu

Type of Privileges	Requirement		What Can You Do?
Basic	Vascular fellowship		Basic techniques. Arteriography, ballon angioplasty, stents
Advanced	Arteriograms	200	All endo techniques, exclusive
	Interventions	100	of renal stents, AAA stent-grafts, carotid arteriography, and carotid stents
Special	Renal PTA/stent	10	Renal angioplasty and stents
	Stent-graft AAA	10	Stent-grafting of AAA
	Carotid arteriogram	40	Carotid arteriograms
	Carotid stent	10	Carotid stents

Abbreviations: AAA, Abdominal aortic aneurysm; *PTA,* percutaneous transluminal angioplasty.

TABLE 3.
Vascular Specialists Face Competition for Both Open
Vascular and Endovascular Cases

Endovascular Surgery	Open Vascular Surgery
Vascular surgeon	Vascular surgeon
Cardiologist	Cardiothoracic surgeon
Interventional radiologist	General surgeon
Neurointerventional radiologist	Neurosurgeon

tions and communities is that regardless of the endovascular training and or experience of a vascular surgeon, there is often an underlying sense that vascular surgeons are not qualified to perform these procedures. Since there is no exclusive domain for any vascular procedure, vascular surgeons are used to competing with many specialists for both open and endovascular surgery (Table 3). The one important difference between vascular surgeons and others who would like to include the vascular system in their work is that vascular surgery is the only specialty that can provide the entire spectrum of care. To the extent that vascular surgeons are able to master and deliver all therapeutic approaches, we fulfill our responsibility to the patients for complete vascular care. This requires that we are well versed in endovascular techniques amongst other things. To the extent that we abdicate this responsibility to other disciplines, the future of vascular surgery as a specialty could be jeopardized.

PLANNING FOR AND OBTAINING EQUIPMENT

To perform endovascular cases, a surgeon must have a place to work. There are 3 popular options: (1) perform endovascular procedures in the operating room using portable fluoroscopic equipment; (2) perform procedures in an angio suite; or (3) construct an endovascular operating room where procedures may be percutaneous, open, or combined.[21-23]

Almost all endovascular procedures can be performed with a portable digital fluoroscopic unit that is now available in most operating rooms. However, portable units are cumbersome, low power, and add time to the procedure. They are useful for helping a surgeon start a program, but c-arms have limitations when attempting to expand an endovascular practice. A stationary fluoroscopic unit confers multiple advantages that will significantly enhance an endovascular practice. The advantages and disadvantages of these 2 methods of imaging are compared in Table 4. The vascular specialist should early on have a plan for how access to fixed imaging equipment will be obtained. An institution would never bring a cardiologist on staff without the availability of more than $1 million of imaging equipment. The days when vascular surgeons can perform their work with simple arterial clamps and suture material are over. To practice as a vascular specialist, advanced imaging equipment is required!

PROCURING AND MAINTAINING ENDOVASCULAR INVENTORY

The inventory that is available to the vascular specialist is every bit as important as the endovascular skills that must be obtained to use this inventory. The supplies and devices that a specialist uses to accomplish daily practice help to define who that specialist is and what the specialist's scope of practice includes. To offer a full spectrum of vascular care, the tools of the trade must be available. The availability of various choices for guidewires, catheters, stents, and other supplies is absolutely essential. Any complex endovascular procedure, such as a multistent iliac reconstruction or a renal or carotid stent, can be hindered or facilitated by the various inventory choices available. Tips for developing and maintaining an endovascular inventory are listed in Table 5. Vascular specialists must be clear and specific about what they need to treat patients.

An endovascular inventory is subject to much more change than a standard operating room inventory for open surgery. New supplies are introduced on a regular basis. It is the vascular specialist's responsibility to request new supplies, be aware of the location of each of the various devices, and update the inventory. Borrowing catheters, supplies, and stents from another location when performing

---

TABLE 4.
Stationary Versus Portable Fluoroscopic Imaging Equipment

	Stationary	Portable
Advantages	Better resolution	Less expensive
	Easy to use	Can be used in different locations
	Versatile positioning	Best units available simulate quality
	Bolus chase	of stationary equipment-resolution,
		road mapping, post-image
		processing, storage
Disadvantages	More expensive	Inconvenient and cumbersome
	Usage restricted to single location	to move and position
	Some units difficult to adapt to	Resolution inferior to fixed unit
	use with open surgery	Impractical for survey arteriography
	Requires room renovation	Often no dedicated personnel

(Courtesy of Schneider PA: *Endovascular Skills*. New York, Marcel Dekker, Inc, 2003, p 177.)

TABLE 5.

Tips for Developing and Maintaining an Endovascular Inventory

- Copy a colleague's inventory—borrow the "list," always check the closet when you visit
- Pick 2 or 3 companies based upon service and quality
- Check catalogues—lots of competing products can be compared
- Know your reps—they know the most about what people are using
- Read materials and methods—see what others use for complex cases
- Use a case card approach—develop your own, be clear about what you need
- Put someone in charge of inventory—reordering disposables, keep it organized
- Update on a regular basis—order new items as they become available

(Modified from Schneider PA: *Endovascular Skills.* New York, Marcel Dekker, Inc, 2003, p 350.)

---

procedures in the operating room is illogical and harmful to patients. The likelihood of making it halfway through a case and not having what you need is high. A free-standing inventory must be available wherever the specialist is planning to work.

A basic inventory of access sheaths, flush and selective catheters, and guidewires must be obtained. After that, inventory accumulates more gradually, usually by ordering a set of supplies for each new procedure. Endovascular procedures should be performed by using a "case card" approach so that the circulating nursing and technical personnel are well aware ahead of time which equipment might be needed. This inventory can be pulled and made available, and opened as appropriate. Case cards are used routinely for open cases, and yet the tendency with endovascular cases is to pull the needed supplies "one at a time" during the procedure. The "one at a time" approach is inefficient, and occasionally the required device has run out and is not available when it is needed most. An example of a case card for renal artery intervention is shown in Table 6. Case cards can be made up at the surgeon's discretion for any endovascular procedure. The inventory should be stored on rolling carts that can be moved from one place to another, allowing close proximity to the ongoing endovascular procedure.

Trying to perform endovascular procedures without a wide variety of choices is setting yourself up for failure. Endovascular surgery differs from open surgery in that it is common to try one catheter or tool and have it not work, go on to the second and third, and sometimes fourth choice. The range of choices and options with open surgery is smaller once the case has started. Since endovascular surgery has been incorporated in various degrees into the treatment of vascular problems, it is not unusual for an endovascular surgeon to be assisted by an operating staff that has little experience with endovascular techniques, and little understanding of endovascular inventory. The endovascular surgeon must take the initiative to orient the staff, frequently reevaluate the availability of new potential inventory items, and to be aware of the inventory items that may be used in given situations.[24]

ESTABLISHING THE SCOPE OF PRACTICE

What is the scope of your endovascular program? Who will be performing endovascular surgery? Will there be nonvascular specialists in your program? What is the proficiency level you hope to obtain? Does the program have a facility that is equipped to combine endovascular and open procedures? Is the program limited to abdominal aortic aneurysm stent-grafting? Will the full range of occlusive disease be treated, including carotid, renal, and tibial disease? Is there an opportunity to include venous disease? Will thrombolytic therapy, closure devices, and advanced endovascular techniques be used? Will carbon dioxide and gadolinium arteriography be available? Is the hospital's administration supportive of your program?

TABLE 6.
"Case Card" for Renal Artery Intervention

Guidewire	Starting guidewire	Bentson	145-cm length	0.035 in. in diameter
	Selective guidewire	Magic Torque	180 cm	0.035 in. (marker tip)
		Glidewire	180 cm	0.035 in (angled tip)
	Exchange guidewire	Rosen	180 cm	0.035 in. (J tip)
Catheter	Flush catheter	Omni-flush	65-cm length	5 Fr
	Selective catheter	Cobra C_1, C_2	65, 80	5 Fr
		Renal double curve	65, 80	5 Fr
		Renal curve 1, 2	65, 80	5 Fr
		SOS omni 2	80	5 Fr
Sheath	Selective guide sheath	Ansel 1, 2, 3	45-cm length	6 Fr, 7 Fr
		RDC	55 cm	7 Fr
Balloon	Balloon angioplasty catheter	Balloon diameter	4, 5, 6, 7 mm	5 Fr
		Balloon length	2, 4 cm	
		Catheter shaft	75 cm length	
Stent*	Balloon-expandable stent	Palmaz-Corinthian or Genesis (premounted)	Stent diameter Stent length Shaft length	5, 6, 7 mm 12-29 mm 80 cm

*No stents are approved by the FDA for routine usage in this vascular bed.
(Courtesy of Schneider PA: *Endovascular Skills*. New York, Marcel Dekker, Inc, 2003, p 284.)

Not all of these issues need to be decided ahead of time, but one ought to take the opportunity to consider the full scope of endovascular possibilities in setting up the program. The answers to these questions have implications with respect to endovascular skills, imaging equipment, and inventory. Any procedures you decide not to include in your program will probably be performed by someone else; if not at the present time, then in the future, and if not in your institution, then the patients will be referred to other institutions. Provided that the appropriate levels of expertise and resources are available, the broader the scope of the program, the higher the likelihood of success.

Endovascular surgery is a dynamic field and is currently in a phase of rapid development. No matter what your current situation might be, if you are treating vascular disease, your program will evolve. Each program should have methods for introducing new technology. This should be discussed on a departmental/divisional level. As new techniques develop, one option is to designate one member of the team to learn these techniques and bring them back to the rest of the group. New techniques are being developed so frequently that it is almost impossible for any one person to spend the time away to learn them all. For example, in our program, one of us has developed extra facility with aortic aneurysm stent-grafts and is primarily responsible for evaluating new grafts as they become available. Another one of us has pursued carotid stenting and evaluation of distal protection devices, and has coordinated our participation in carotid stent trials. Another of us has focused on alternative contrast agents, including carbon dioxide and gadolinium, and mechanical thrombectomy devices. As these new techniques are incorporated into our armamentarium, each of us eventually gains expertise.

UNDERSTANDING THE MARKET FOR ENDOVASCULAR PROCEDURES

Where will the cases come from? How can endovascular techniques be introduced into current practice? How can endovascular procedures contribute to the marketing of vascular services?

Every busy vascular practice includes many opportunities for fluoroscopic imaging and endovascular intervention as a complement to current caseload. One obvious source of cases is the use of simultaneous combined inflow percutaneous transluminal angioplasty (PTA) or outflow PTA for an open surgical reconstruction. Another option is to proceed with completion arteriography after open surgeries, such as infrainguinal bypass, carotid endarterectomy, revision of a dialysis graft, and others. When acute lower extremity ischemia requires surgery, intraoperative fluoroscopy may be used to guide catheter passage, thrombus extraction, and any endovascular techniques that are required to complement the open surgical procedure. Consider performing noninvasive imaging with duplex mapping, magnetic resonance angiography, or both, before elective lower extremity revascularization for chronic ischemia. Subsequently, confirmatory arteriography can be performed in the operating room before reconstruction. In addition, endovascular cases may be referred by other surgeons who may want to gain additional experience by participating in the procedure. When a surgeon becomes oriented to the potential of endovascular techniques, there are many opportunities to integrate these techniques into the standard vascular surgery practice.

It turns out that what is best for vascular surgery is also best for patients: we need to offer *complete* vascular care. There is currently a significant effort in every area of surgery to convert to less invasive interventions to improve outcomes and decrease morbidity. For patients to receive optimal care, the vascular specialist must be able to deliver a complete spectrum of treatment options, and endovascular is one of these. Patients and referring physicians need to know that the less invasive options are being considered and performed by the vascular service. The old image of the vascular surgeon as the one who is obligated to the scalpel and the doubter of new technology is counterproductive. We need to be able to consider judiciously and without prejudice all the available approaches, and let the patients decide what they want.

HANDLING INSTITUTIONAL POLITICS

Virtually all vascular surgeons who have embraced these techniques have had to compete for the right to perform catheter-based techniques in their practices. Many surgeons have been forced to limit their endovascular practices or make compromises to get along in their institutions, that are not in the best interest of patient care. Unfortunately, nonproductive and even acrimonious situations have been common. Given that vascular surgeons are often responsible for primary vascular care, it may seem somewhat ironic that we face so much resistance when we attempt to use developing technology and medical knowledge to benefit patient care.

No one has all the right answers for this, and each institution seems to have evolved into its own way. A key factor in maneuvering one's way through potentially very difficult and contentious institutional politics is to stay focused on the patient. Set high standards and go about meeting them. Rely on external standards to the extent that this is possible. A modern and sustainable vascular practice cannot be shaped around what physicians in other nonvascular disciplines expect. Develop the practice around what is best for your patients and what you would want for your parents. In addition, it is absolutely essential that the vascular surgeon makes it clear that endovascular surgery is within the scope of vascular practice.

A major complaint among vascular surgeons is that they are excluded from endovascular intervention. Since endovascular interventions can be performed in the operating room, even if access to an angiographic suite or cardiac laboratory is not an option, an endovascular program can be begun without addressing certain territorial issues. Portable imaging equipment is not optimal, but it has been shown to be adequate for many of the most complex endovascular cases performed, including carotid stents, abdominal aortic stent-grafting, embolization of endoleaks, and complex lower extremity reconstructions. At the same time, a successful program will eventually require that the surgeon gains access to fixed imaging equipment and a suite.

Endovascular skills are frequently introduced by a junior member of the division/department. It must be recognized, however, that the newest department member is unlikely to have the political clout to effect real change. Introducing endovascular procedures into the surgeon's portfolio often requires a joint and coordinated effort by junior and senior staff.

ASSESSING OUTCOMES

Endovascular therapy can provide a less morbid solution for otherwise complex problems. The morbidity must be lower than for open repair, and the durability must at least be acceptable for the given patient population. Although endovascular procedures are not generally as durable as open procedures, the long-term survival of the vascular population is diminished by cardiovascular and neoplastic disease. In some patients, a less morbid and durable procedure may be preferable to a longer lasting but more aggressive intervention. Outcomes for endovascular procedures are just as important as for open procedures. Understanding the overall outcomes of endovascular interventions helps the surgeon to better decide how to select the best treatment for each patient. Surgeons have always been most interested in follow-up and long-term outcomes, and this philosophy should not change as we learn to perform endovascular techniques.

VASCULAR AT KAISER HAWAII

The Division of Vascular Therapy at Kaiser Hawaii includes 3 full-time vascular surgeons, a physician assistant, an accredited vascular laboratory, and an endovascular operating room. We manage the vascular needs of approximately 240,000 Hawaii residents. Endovascular cases have steadily grown as a proportion of our program; 3% in 1992, 26% in 1997, 50% in 2001, and more than half currently. Over the past 5 years, the volume of cases increased by 39%, but the number of open cases peaked in 2001 and is decreasing. Along with continued increases in volume, the trend toward a greater percentage of cases being performed with endovascular approaches will continue for the foreseeable future. The number of open cases will likely decrease as it has for others.[5,25,26] We anticipate that endovascular techniques will continue to develop until it is the treatment of choice for most conditions, with open surgery

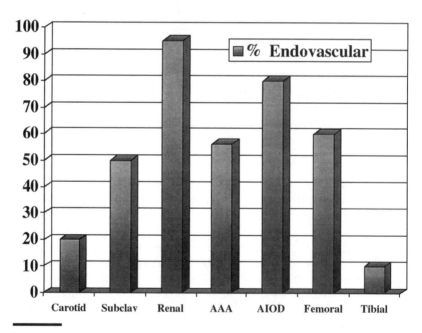

FIGURE 1.

Kaiser Hawaii percentage of cases performed using endovascular surgery in various vascular beds in 2002, including extracranial carotid occlusive disease *(carotid)*, subclavian occlusive disease *(subclav)*, renovascular disease *(renal)*, abdominal aortic aneurysm *(AAA)*, aortoiliac occlusive disease *(AIOD)*, femoral-popliteal disease *(femoral)*, and infrapopliteal disease *(tibial)*.

being necessary for patients who have experienced endovascular failure. The percentage of cases in our program that were performed with endovascular techniques in the various vascular beds in 2002 is shown in Figure 1.

We expect that endovascular techniques will continue to increase in percentage in both the carotid and tibial beds over the next several years as techniques and skills improve in these areas. Other areas that are likely to grow over the next few years are new stent-grafts including a thoracic device and stent-grafts with suprarenal fixation and side branch technology; endovascular treatment of aortic dissection; and thrombolysis for acute lower extremity deep vein thrombosis. Our plan is to continue to incorporate new techniques into our practice as they are developed.

THE FUTURE OF ENDOVASCULAR, OR WHY YOU OUGHT TO START A PROGRAM TODAY

1. The need for those who only perform open surgery is at the present time limited and is likely to diminish significantly over the next 5 to 10 years.
2. Open vascular surgery is not likely to be developed much further and will never again be the mainstay treatment for vascular disease. Open surgery will be replaced or at least become substantially less important. If we want to treat vascular disease, we must have all the options within our armamentarium. To do less would be a disservice to the patients.
3. Although some persons don't agree, including a number of vascular surgeons, that endovascular will become the mainstay of treatment, realize that problems arising with endovascular procedures will almost always be solved with the further development of new endovascular techniques.
4. Carotid, renal, and infrapopliteal occlusive disease is more readily treatable with balloon angioplasty and stent after the development of lower profile angioplasty systems using 0.014-inch wires. A wide variety of stents are now available and can be used to treat vascular disease in virtually every vascular bed.
5. Once endovascular therapy has been integrated into the culture of the vascular surgeon, there is no turning back. New tools, such as drug-eluting stents, covered stents, intraluminal cutters, better closure devices, and advanced recanalization drugs and devices, are under development and will help to shape the future treatment of vascular disease.

REFERENCES

1. Schneider PA, Silva MB: Initiating a program in carotid stenting, in Pearce WH, Matsumura JS, Yao JST (eds): *Trends in Vascular Surgery.* Chicago, Precept Press, pp 121-135, 2004.
2. Messina LM, Schneider DB, Chuter TA, et al: Integrated fellowship in vascular surgery and interventional radiology: A new paradigm in vascular training. *Ann Surg* 236:408-414, 2002.
3. Veith FJ, Sanchez LA, Ohki T: Should vascular surgeons perform endovascular procedures and how can they acquire the skills to do so? *Semin Vasc Surg* 10:191-196, 1997.
4. Sanders J: Development and implementation of an endovascular surgery program in a community general hospital. *J Healthc Manag* 47: 3335-3340, 2002.
5. Sullivan TM, Taylor SM, Blackhurst DW, et al: Has endovascular surgery reduced the number of open vascular operations performed by an established surgical practice? *J Vasc Surg* 36:514-519, 2002.
6. Schneider PA: Endovascular concepts, in Schneider PA (ed): *Endovascular Skills.* New York, Marcel Dekker, 2003, pp 1-4.
7. Katzen BT: The future of catheter-based angiography: Implications for the vascular interventionalist. *Radiol Clin North Am* 40:689-692, 2002.
8. Schneider PA, Ogawa DY, Rush MR: Lower extremity revasularization without contrast arteriography: Operation based upon duplex is feasible. *Cardiovasc Surg* 7:699-703, 1999.
9. Ahn SS, Moore WS (eds): *Endovascular Surgery.* Philadelphia, WB Saunders, 2001.
10. Kim D, Orron DE (eds): *Peripheral Vascular Imaging and Intervention.* St Louis, Mosby, 1992.
11. Schneider PA: *Endovascular Skills.* New York, Marcel Dekker, 2003.
12. Hodgson KJ, Mattos MA, Mansour A, et al: Incorporation of endovascular training into a vascular fellowship program. *Am J Surg* 170:168-173, 1995.
13. Silva MB, Hobson RW, Jamil Z, et al: A program of operative angioplasty: Endovascular intervention and the vascular surgeon. *J Vasc Surg* 24: 963-971, 1996.
14. Kashyap VS, Ahn SS, Davis MR, et al: Trends in vascular surgery training. *J Endovasc Ther* 9:633-638, 2002.
15. White RA, Hodgson KJ, Ahn SS, et al: Endovascular interventions training and credentialing for vascular surgeons. *J Vasc Surg* 29:177-186, 1999.
16. Levin DC, Becker GJ, Dorros G, et al: Training standards for physicians performing peripheral angioplasty and other percutaneous peripheral vascular interventions: A statement for health professions from the Special Writing Group of the Councils on Cardiovascular Radiology, Cardio-Thoracic and Vascular Surgery, and Clinical Cardiology, the American Heart Association. *Circulation* 86:1348-1350, 1992.

17. Lewis CA, Sacks D, Cardella JF, et al: Position statement: Documenting physician experience for credentials for peripheral arterial procedures: What you need to know. *J Vasc Interv Radiol* 13:453-454, 2002.

18. Sacks D, Becker GJ, Matalon TAS: Credentials for peripheral angioplasty: Comments on Society of Cardiac Angiography and Intervention Revisions. *J Vasc Interv Radiol* 12:277-280, 2001.

19. Spies JB, Bakal CW, Burke DR, et al: Standards for interventional radiology: Standards of Practice Committee of the SCVIR. *J Vasc Interv Radiol* 2:59-65, 1991.

20. Spittell JA, Nanda GC, Creager MA, et al: Recommendations for peripheral transluminal angioplasty training and facilities. ACC Peripheral Vascular Disease Committee. *J Am Coll Cardiol* 21:546-548, 1993.

21. Dietrich EB: Endovascular suite design, in White RA, Fogarty TJ (eds): *Peripheral Endovascular Interventions*. St Louis, Mosby, 1996, pp 129-139.

22. Mansour MA, Hodgson KJ: Preparing the endovascular operating room suite, in Moore WS, Ahn SS (eds): *Endovascular Surgery*. Philadelphia, WB Saunders, 2001, pp 3-13.

23. Schneider PA: Where do we work? in Schneider PA (ed): *Endovascular Skills*. New York, Marcel Dekker, 2003, pp 175-181.

24. Schneider PA, Caps MT: Essential operating room equipment, personnel, and catheter inventory for endovascular repair of abdominal aortic aneurysms, in Hakaim AG (ed): *Current Endovascular Treatment of Abdominal Aortic Aneurysms*. New York, Futura Press, in press.

25. Lin PH, Bush RL, Milas M, et al: Impact of an endovascular program on the operative experience of abdominal aortic aneurysm in vascular fellowship and general surgery residency. *Am J Surg* 186:189-193, 2003.

26. Choi ET, Wyble CW, Rubin BG, et al: Evolution of vascular fellowship training in the new era of endovascular techniques. *J Vasc Surg* 33: S106-S110, 2001.

CHAPTER 3

Current Indications for Carotid Angioplasty and Stent: What Is the Future?

Neal C. Hadro
New York-Presbyterian Hospital, New York, NY

Daniel G. Clair, MD
Vice Chairman, Department of Vascular Surgery, Cleveland Clinic
Foundation

Stroke prevention continues to challenge the best efforts of modern multidisciplinary medicine. Stroke not only ranks as the third leading cause of death behind heart disease and cancer, but stroke additionally exacts a substantial cost on society in the form of disability and the expense of long-term care.[1] Extracranial carotid occlusive disease is estimated to be responsible for stroke in approximately one third of patients who have a cerebrovascular event.[2] This prevalence underscores the importance of optimizing treatment strategies to prevent patients with carotid occlusive disease from developing the morbidity and mortality that elevates stroke to its preeminent level as a major public health problem.

As a prelude to defining a role for carotid angioplasty and stenting (CAS), it is essential to briefly revisit the history of open carotid revascularization. The history of carotid surgery depicts a methodical journey to legitimacy of a technique that has the same goal as carotid stenting. This history can therefore serve a dual purpose. First, results of carotid endarterectomy (CEA) can be compared with data gained from contemporary trials of CAS. Also, mistakes made in trials of CEA should be avoided when designing evaluations of carotid stenting.

Surgical therapy for extracranial carotid occlusive disease was first described in the 1950s.[3] In the early to mid 1990s, the results of

2 major prospective randomized trials, the North American Symptomatic Carotid Endarterectomy Trial (NASCET) and the Asymptomatic Carotid Atherosclerosis Study (ACAS), were reported.[4,5] These landmark studies validated the role of surgical therapy performed by selected providers to prevent stroke in certain cohorts of symptomatic and asymptomatic patients. The release of these results initiated a significant increase in the number of CEAs performed annually in communities throughout the nation.[6,7] Yet, despite the findings of these multicentered trials, design restrictions continue to invite criticism about the global application of their results to the community at large. Surgeons in ACAS and NASCET were experienced, whereas surgeons in the community may not have sufficient volume to achieve these same excellent results.[6-13] Moreover, many higher risk patients who are currently treated with CEA were excluded from these large trials because of age and medical comorbidities. Thus, the definitive management of carotid disease for all patients encountered in clinical practice continues to be a work in progress, since it appears that the outcomes of CEA in many community and tertiary centers are not truly representative of what was achieved in NASCET- or ACAS-eligible patients.[14-18] These factors make a comparison of CEA with contemporary carotid stenting somewhat difficult. For example, the recent reported results for carotid stenting from the Sapphire trial are in a cohort of high-risk patients. It is impossible to compare findings from this study with those of ACAS or NASCET.

PROCEDURE

CAS techniques have been refined since the late 1990s.[19-21] The technique is well described, and the following is a brief summary of the technical details of the procedure. Before the procedure, the patient is begun on aggressive antiplatelet therapy, including aspirin and clopidogrel. Preparation in the room before the procedure is as important as the technique used during the procedure. One should have available a number of vasoactive medications, including intravenous infusions of nitroglycerin, nitroprusside, and neosynephrine for use in response to hemodynamic instability. Medications such as atropine for bradycardia and dopamine should also be easily accessible. Support staff needs to be readily able to quickly treat hypotension or hypertension or bradycardia. β-Blockers are generally avoided so as not to worsen the bradycardia that can result from dilatation of the carotid bulb. Large-bore intravenous access is required should volume need to be rapidly infused. A method of assessing adequacy of anticoagulation is also needed in proximity to the procedural area. The optimal method of evaluating anticoagulation is via measurement of activated clotting times. Suction, oxygen, continuous electrocardiographic monitoring, measurement of oxygen saturation, and arterial pressure monitoring are essential. Adequate imaging is imperative as well. One should have an imaging system that allows rotation from an anterior-posterior to a full lateral view so that optimal interrogation of all vessels can be achieved.

Access is obtained most often via the femoral artery by using a Seldinger technique followed by placement of either a 5F or 6F sheath. Subsequently, a flush catheter is placed into the aortic arch for diagnostic arch arteriography. This view is best performed in the left anterior oblique projection, to help isolate the origins of the great vessels from the aortic arch. A left anterior oblique projection of 30° to 60° should be used, depending on the rotation of the aorta in the chest. One should attempt to obtain the broadest view of the arch allowing the greatest separation of the origins of the great vessels. Rotating the image-intensifier so that the flush catheter's curve is maximally flattened helps to optimize the profile of the origins of the great vessels. This aids in subsequent individual selection of arch vessels. The patient is adequately heparinized to maintain an activated clotting time greater than 250 seconds. This parameter is checked frequently, and arterial pressure is monitored continuously. Selective access to the common carotid arteries is best achieved with the least angled catheter possible. The advantage of using a less angled catheter becomes obvious when one advances this catheter over the wire used to cannulate the common carotid artery. Reversed curve catheters, such as the Simmons or Vitek, can be difficult to advance into the carotid artery. These catheters, however, have their advantages, particularly when cannulating the left common carotid artery. Depending on the necessary information to be gained, one may choose to perform a full 4-vessel cerebral angiogram or merely to image the vessel in question. The technique of cerebral angiography will not be reviewed here. After selection of the vessel to be treated, the catheter is advanced into the base of the vessel to allow procurement of a diagnostic image of the carotid bifurcation and the intracerebral vessels. A standard series of anteroposterior, lateral, and oblique cervical views are obtained, with attention to profiling the carotid bifurcation to best elucidate the area of stenosis. In addition, anteroposterior and lateral cerebral views should be obtained to determine baseline cerebral vascular anatomy. The cerebral views are essential and allow identification of intracranial pathology as well as cerebral cross-filling. The latter is of importance if an occlusion balloon is to be used during the procedure for distal cerebral protection. These intracranial images also serve as a baseline for comparison, should an adverse neurologic event occur and intracranial rescue be necessary.

After the diagnostic portion of the procedure, attention is focused on the index lesion that requires treatment. A roadmap angiogram is performed, and a hydrophilic wire is advanced into the external carotid artery followed by the catheter. The hydrophilic wire is removed and replaced with a stiff wire (Amplatz super-stiff 0.035-inch wire, Boston Scientific, Natick, Mass). This rigid wire will allow exchange of the diagnostic catheter for a 6F sheath through which the revascularization procedure will be performed. Alternatively, an 8F guide catheter can be used in conjunction with a 5F or 6F diagnostic catheter to gain access to the common carotid artery. The guide technique results in a larger groin puncture, but a guide is useful for more challenging arch anatomy. A guide can traverse complex anatomy that may be difficult to navigate with a more flexible sheath.

With either a 6F sheath or an 8F guide situated in the common carotid artery, another angiographic roadmap is obtained of the bifurcation, and a protection device, such as a filter wire or occlusion balloon, is advanced beyond the lesion. Depending on the protection device selected, additional images are acquired to verify appropriate apposition of the device against the vessel wall or completeness of occlusion with an occlusion balloon. Placement of the protection device may require "pre" predilation with a 2-mm balloon, or use of a .014 or .018 "buddy wire" if the stenosis is high grade or if the anatomy is difficult. The area of stenosis should most often be predilated before traversing the lesion with the delivery device for the stent. The patient is frequently pretreated with 0.5 mg of atropine to prevent a bradycardic response during bulb dilation. A slightly longer balloon system should be used to ensure that the lesion is completely treated with a single inflation. A balloon diameter of 4 mm should allow passage of nearly any self-expanding stent delivery system. A self-expanding stent is then placed into position, and the adequacy of coverage is confirmed by imaging. Ideally, this imaging should be performed without subtraction if possible. The advantage of this approach is that the stent position relative to the arterial anatomy is not altered, as can happen during a deep inspiration that is required for acquisition of a subtraction image. Pre–stent deployment imaging can be difficult, if not impossible, in the setting of an occlusion balloon. A self-expanding stent is preferable to a balloon-mounted stent. A self-expanding stent lessens the hemodynamic effects of stent placement, since the bulb is not overdilated.

Also, there remains a risk of extrinsic compression in balloon-mounted stents.[22] The stent is deployed to cover the entire internal carotid artery lesion, and if necessary, the stent should be extended into the common carotid artery. Frequently, the origin of the external carotid artery is covered, which is acceptable. Lastly, the stent is postdilated to an appropriate profile, often 5 to 6 mm, and a completion carotid and cerebral arteriogram is performed after the distal protection device is removed.

MAJOR STUDIES, REGISTRIES, AND MINOR SERIES

Carotid angioplasty was initially described in the early 1980s and was used for the treatment of fibromuscular dysplasia, atherosclerotic lesions, and recurrent carotid arterial stenoses.[23-26] As early as 1986, a review of 94 patients was reported in the literature.[27] As further experience with this technique was gained, stenting became more routine, and in the late 1990s, a number of individual cases and several small series were reported.[20,21] The outcomes of some of these early trials were unfavorable compared with CEA. These poor outcomes were likely related to inappropriate patient selection, a steep learning curve, and technology in its infancy. The major contemporary trials and registries outlined below are remarkable for their large patient numbers and consistent demonstration of the viability of this procedure. Many smaller trials are available in which newly developed stents or protection systems, new-generation antiplatelet agents, or specific demographic groups (eg, octogenarians, restenosis, and irradiated necks) have been evaluated. While many of these trials have been criticized for having too few patients, being retrospective, or lacking unmatched controls, they are similar in methodology to the large body of retrospective literature, which serves as the impetus for expanding the indications of CEA beyond NASCET, ACAS, or both. At a minimum, the consistently reproducible and safe outcomes of CAS provide sufficient evidence to encourage enrollment of patients into prospective trials comparing CEA with CAS.

There are currently 3 completed randomized trials comparing CAS with CEA. The first completed trial is the Carotid and Vertebral Artery Transluminal Angioplasty Study (CAVATAS), which was presented in 2001.[28] In this multicenter trial, 504 patients were randomly assigned to either endovascular or surgical treatment for significant carotid stenosis. Patients were enrolled in 22 centers in Europe. There were no age limits, but there were anatomic exclusion criteria. Patients were excluded if they were not candidates for surgical revascularization for either anatomic or physiologic reasons.

As well, patients with thrombus within the carotid artery and those with severe tortuosity thought to contraindicate percutaneous revascularization were also excluded. The study began in March 1992, and the use of stents was allowed from 1994 onward. The specific techniques of surgical and percutaneous revascularization were left up to the interventionalists. Only 26% of the endovascular patients received a stent, with the majority receiving primary angioplasty alone. Cerebral protection devices were not available. The patients were followed up for 3 years, and an independent neurologist evaluated each patient. The rates of disabling stroke in the surgical and endovascular groups were similar (4% surgical vs 4% endovascular). There was also no difference in the mortality rate or rate of nondisabling stroke (mortality, 2% surgical vs 3% endovascular; stroke, 4% surgical vs 4% endovascular). Similar outcomes were also noted for the composite end point of any stroke or death within 30 days (9.9% surgical vs 10% endovascular). Cranial nerve injury (8.7%) and neck hematoma (6.7%) were significantly higher in surgical patients, with a low incidence of groin hematoma (1.7%) and no cranial nerve injuries in endovascular patients. At 1 year, the restenosis rate was higher in the endovascular group, but over 3 years, the stroke rate was equivalent. This study was thought to be significant in that it demonstrated similar outcomes for CEA and CAS. The morbidity and mortality of both groups, however, was high. Of note, only a minority of endovascular patients received stents after angioplasty, perhaps explaining the increased incidence of restenosis in the angioplasty cohort, and no cerebral protection was used. As will be discussed later, there are overwhelming data to support the benefit of stents and protective devices in endoluminal treatment of carotid stenosis.

A smaller, community hospital–based randomized trial comparing endarterectomy to angioplasty and stenting was recently reported.[29] In this trial, 104 symptomatic patients with greater than 70% carotid stenosis were randomly assigned to undergo either surgical or percutaneous revascularization. In the absence of cerebral protection, and using the Wallstent (Boston Scientific), these investigators noted no differences in major adverse events (death, stroke, and transient ischemic attack) between the 2 groups. There was a single mortality in the surgical group and one transient ischemic attack in the endovascular group, and no other major adverse events occurred. Although the number of patients was small, the trial impressively demonstrated that carotid stenting can be safely performed in a community hospital.

The last completed randomized trial is Stenting and Angioplasty with Protection in Patients at High-risk for Endarterectomy (SAPPHIRE), which at the time this chapter was written has been published only in abstract form.[30] Investigators randomly assigned asymptomatic patients with greater than 80% stenosis and symptomatic patients with greater than 50% stenosis who were deemed "high risk" based on a predetermined list of anatomic and physiologic risk categories. Patients subsequently underwent either surgical revascularization or percutaneous revascularization with a filter protection device (Angioguard, Cordis, Johnson & Johnson, Warren, NJ). A stent registry was available for patients who were thought to be at prohibitive risk for CEA. All patients were evaluated by a neurologist before and after the procedure. Major adverse events were defined as death, any stroke, or myocardial infarction (Q wave or non-Q wave), and these were assessed at 30 days and then at 1 year. Overall, 307 patients underwent randomization. There were no differences between the 2 groups when major adverse events were individually assessed. However, there was an advantage for patients undergoing percutaneous intervention when the composite end point of death, any stroke, or myocardial infarction was assessed (5.8% intervention vs 12.6% surgery). Critical evaluation of this trial awaits formal publication of the data; however, the addition of myocardial infarction as a major end point is radically different from any other study that has been previously performed to evaluate the treatment of carotid artery stenosis. Despite controversy about the inclusion of coronary events, this trial demonstrated for high-risk patients that at minimum, the outcomes for the 2 procedures are similar. Thus, it would appear that there are certain high-risk patients for whom an interventional approach is advisable. Should acute coronary events be a predictor of long-term cardiovascular death (and there is some evidence to suggest this to be the case), the inclusion of this end point may be an additional important advantage for high-risk patients treated with an endovascular approach. Criticisms of this study include the high percentage of asymptomatic patients who were included and the relatively high stroke and death rate for these asymptomatic patients compared with that of ACAS (4.5% endovascular vs 6.6% surgery; $P = $ not significant). While it is true these numbers are higher than those published in the ACAS trial, it has become evident that SAPPHIRE studied a different patient population than ACAS, and direct comparisons clearly are not applicable between the 2 groups. These 3 trials present compelling evidence for the need to proceed with a thorough comparison of CAS and CEA in a larger and more diverse cohort of patients.

Nonrandomized results of CAS have been reported by multiple investigators. Wholey et al[31,32] recently reported the results of a multicenter registry of CAS. Inclusive were the outcomes of more than 12,000 carotid interventions at 53 centers. Technical success of stent placement was achieved in 98.9% of patients. The 30-day risk of any stroke and death was 4.0%, with a major stroke rate of 1.2% and a mortality rate of 0.6%. The authors further evaluated the outcomes of procedures performed with and without cerebral protection in symptomatic and asymptomatic patients. There was a statistically significant advantage of protection when performed in symptomatic (6.0% unprotected vs 2.7% protected; $P < .0001$) and asymptomatic (4.0% unprotected vs 1.8% protected; $P < .0001$) patients. More than 2000 procedures were performed in asymptomatic patients using protection; the combined stroke and death rate of 1.8% is similar to what might be anticipated with a series of surgical endarterectomy in a similar population. This study is obviously subject to the limitations of any registry; however, results from this registry over time are clearly improving, and it appears that outcomes are approaching those of CEA.

The ongoing Carotid Revascularization Endarterectomy versus Stent Trial (CREST) aims to compare endarterectomy versus angioplasty and stenting for symptomatic lesions in "low-risk" or NASCET-eligible patients.[33] This is a well-designed trial that puts surgery and endarterectomy head to head on a level playing field. Given the low overall event rate in this well-selected group, it is anticipated, however, that 2500 patients will need to be enrolled in 40 centers to develop meaningful comparisons.[34,35] Given that many open surgical patients in any individual surgeon's practice are not NASCET eligible and also that enrollment is predicated on surgeons referring low-risk patients away from surgery, the goal of enrollment is hopefully not overly ambitious.

In addition to these studies, there are many retrospective, nonrandomized reports where specific variables such as age, rate of restenosis, or identifiable risk factors have been isolated. There are also several prospective evaluations of investigational devices such as new stents or cerebral protection devices currently underway. Although the usefulness of these types of series is limited, it is remarkable to note the consistently reproducible technical success rates and the generally low rate of complications across all studies, and their favorable comparison with similarly designed surgical series.

One of the earliest patient cohorts identified as appropriate for CAS is patients with recurrent stenosis from prior endarterectomy. Despite isolated reports of superb results with reoperative endarterectomy,[36] reoperative carotid surgery is associated with an increased incidence of cranial nerve injury and stroke. The smooth nonulcerated surface provided by intimal hyperplasia with its low risk of embolization makes these patients intuitively attractive candidates for angioplasty and stenting. In 1996, Yadav et al[37] presented a series of 22 patients who underwent angioplasty and stenting for restenosis after CEA. All patients referred for recurrent stenosis were treated with stent, and all procedures were angiographically successful. There was one minor stroke reported in this series (4%), which was an extension of a prior middle cerebral artery stroke. Interestingly, restenosis by angiography developed in 19% of patients at 6 months. A large multicenter registry was presented by New et al[38] in 2000, with 338 patients with restenosis undergoing 358 stenting procedures. The overall 30-day stroke and death rate was 3.7%, a favorable rate when compared with the surgical risk that might be associated with these procedures. The minor stroke rate was 1.7%, the major stroke rate was 0.8%, the fatal stroke rate was 0.3%, and the stroke-related death rate was 0.9%. The overall 3-year rate of freedom from all fatal and nonfatal strokes was 96%.

Another group of patients that may benefit from CAS are those with a history of cervical irradiation, which presents a difficult area to dissect or a "hostile neck" that is a well-recognized challenge to open surgical revascularization. Alric[39] et al, in 2002, presented a series of 21 patients treated with CAS, including 17 with restenosis and 5 with a history of neck irradiation. There were no procedural complications and no neurologic complications during the mean follow-up period of 16.6 months. Al-Mubarak et al[40] described 14 patients treated with stenting for severe radiation-induced carotid stenosis. Technical success was achieved in all patients. One patient had a minor stroke after the procedure but recovered fully in 2 days. No other complications were encountered. There was no evidence of restenosis in 9 patients (64%) at 6-month follow-up.

Patients with advanced age have been cited as another potentially high-risk group that might benefit from a minimally invasive approach to carotid revascularization. Excellent surgical results for octogenarians and equivocal results in matched groups treated with carotid stent have made this indication uncertain. A recent review of open surgery presented by Rockman et al[41] from New York University documented excellent outcomes in a consecutive series of 161 patients older than 80 years, treated with CEA. They found no difference in the rate of preoperative myocardial infarction, stroke, or death between patients older than 80 and those younger than 80 with open surgery. In parallel, age as a determinant of risk for carotid stenting was evaluated by Ahmadi et al[42] in 2002. A group of 111 consecutive patients treated with CAS were stratified into groups older than or younger than 75 years. There were no significant differences in outcome with respect to technical success of the procedure, complications, or neurologic event rate. Despite these favorable results, emerging data from CREST, which at the time of writing of this chapter is not yet published, suggest that for angioplasty and stent, there may be a positive relationship between stroke and age.

While there are ongoing trials that have been designed to evaluate specific stents or newer antiplatelet agents,[43,44] the most significant major advance in CAS has been the cerebral protection devices, which are dealt with elsewhere in this text.[45-48] Embolic events remain a major concern with CAS. The incidence of clinically silent magnetic resonance imaging findings with postprocedure imaging and intraprocedural "hits" on transcranial Doppler is high with endoluminal treatment of the carotid artery.[49] One study in particular demonstrated significant transcranial Doppler activity at the time before and after balloon dilation and stent deployment. In this study, this increased Doppler activity was reduced when cerebral protection was achieved with an occlusion balloon.

Much data remain to be collected on individual devices with respect to the ease of use, complication rates, and clinical efficacy. The rapid evolution of these devices is responsible for many ongoing device-specific trials. Most are consecutive series of high-risk patients and not randomized against an alternative control group, such as no cerebral protection. While the results of these trials will provide more definitive information about which device to use and for which patient protection is most appropriate, the overall risk/benefit ratio seems to favor the routine use of cerebral protection.[50] A more thorough description of devices and outcomes is available in another section of this chapter.

DURABILITY

Surgeons in general have been concerned about carotid stenting because of issues related to long-term patency, especially with the multiple recent reports noting the excellent long-term results of CEA.[51-53] Regardless of the method of performing endarterectomy, remarkably low rates of recurrent stenosis varying from 2.5% to 7.7% over 5 to 10 years can be achieved. There are clearly insufficient data regarding carotid stenting and restenosis, but some reports have addressed this issue.[23,32,54-56] All of these studies reveal rates of restenosis of less than 8% with follow-ups up to 3 to 4 years, but these data should be viewed with some skepticism since they are derived from retrospective evaluation of single-institution experiences or from registries. As well, the usefulness of established ultrasonographic criteria for determining the degree of stenosis in those who have had carotid artery stenting has been called into question. It may well be necessary to develop specific ultrasound criteria for patients who have had carotid artery stents.

SURGEON'S PERSPECTIVE

To date, there have been no prospective randomized trials similar to NASCET or ACAS comparing carotid stenting alone to medical therapy. Clearly, the ability of carotid stenting to significantly prevent stroke and death is assumed by proxy from the benefit of CEA versus medical therapy. Ultimately, we should expect more of carotid stenting than the fact that it merely is comparable in the perioperative period to surgery. Completing the appropriate trials, however, will not be easy. As witnessed with the development of advanced laparoscopy and endograft therapy for aneurysms, consumer demand has become an increasingly powerful broker that interferes with attempts to test hypotheses with the scientific method. It seems that when patients perceive that their recovery will be hastened and a less invasive alternative is available, there is a lack of acceptance on their part of necessary clinical trials. Since a deliberate and methodical journey that includes rigorous well-designed clinical trials is essential to legitimize any new procedure, we as surgeons believe that carotid stenting should not be an exception. Future studies should be designed to clearly identify the specific subgroups of patients who will benefit from this technique when compared against matched controls receiving either surgery or medical therapy. Furthermore, time will help answer questions about the long-term durability of the procedure with respect to restenosis.

Other questions remain to be answered including an appraisal of provider skills that are necessary for interventionalists to gain expertise with carotid stenting. Moreover, we need to understand the role of stenting in patients with limited life expectancy. We must remember lessons from NASCET and ACAS. Not only must the surgeon be good, but the patient must live long enough to derive the benefit of a stroke-free existence. Given the potentially diminished survival of the truly "high-risk" patient, a trial evaluating the necessity of carotid stenting versus medical therapy alone should likely be undertaken in this patient cohort.

Carotid stenting has been advocated for patients who are considered high risk for surgery. However, the true definition of high risk remains elusive. A number of reports have recently suggested that excellent outcomes can be achieved with CEA in high-risk patients.[14-18] Lepore et al[16] reviewed 2 years of patients at a tertiary care hospital and identified 46.2% as NASCET or ACAS ineligible. The stroke death rate was 1.5% for trial-eligible patients and only 3.6% for those ineligible. Although the adverse outcomes were increased in the "trial-ineligible" group, the results still compare favorably with the outcomes of NASCET and ACAS. Gasparis et al[15] performed a similar analysis identifying 29% of 788 consecutive patients as NASCET "high risk" (68% by comorbidity, 28% by anatomy, and 9% by both). In this series, the stroke death rate was 1.3% in the high-risk group versus 1.1% in the low-risk group.

While these and other authors have reported individual institutional or surgeon expertise in treating challenging high-risk patients, results of high-risk carotid stenting registries and the SAPPHIRE trial argue that with multicenter randomization and neurologic oversight, the results of endarterectomy in these patients are not as good as surgeons would like to believe. The SAPPHIRE study, sponsored by Cordis Corporation, is a randomized comparative study of symptomatic or asymptomatic high-risk patients treated with CEA versus stenting. Preliminary findings of this study suggest at least an equivalent rate of stroke and death in patients treated with these 2 techniques. However, the overall event rate for both groups was high, particularly in the asymptomatic patients. Data from this trial have been used to gain at least tentative approval from the Food and Drug Administration for use of the Angioguard (Cordis) cerebral protection device in high-risk patients. Final approval is imminent, and it is anticipated that this device will be available, and carotid stenting for high-risk patients will be covered by insurers within the next few months. Still in debate, however, are definitions of what constitutes high risk as well as the issue of whether at least some high-risk patients might be better served with medical therapy.

CONCLUSIONS

At present, CAS appears to provide an alternative for patients with contraindications to CEA. In future randomized trials of carotid stenting, it would be ideal to stratify patients to accurately evaluate who derives the greatest benefit from this technique. One easily achieved distinction would be to differentiate anatomic high-risk patients from physiologic high-risk individuals. Evaluation of long-term durability awaits the completion of properly designed, randomized, prospective controlled trials, similar in scope and scrutiny to those used to validate open endarterectomy. However, it is my prediction that carotid stenting will perform superbly in these trials. The final challenges will then be to develop useful, patient-centered algorithms that best integrate the strengths of open, percutaneous, and medical therapies such that the maximum number of patients will derive the greatest benefit from data-driven decision making.

Our challenge today as surgeons is to gain access to and training in carotid stenting. There is little doubt that carotid stenting will play a major role in the treatment of patients with carotid stenosis. Surgeons are accustomed to treating this cohort of patients, and to maintain this role, we must gain the necessary skills and ability to perform endoluminal therapy for carotid disease. This is a major challenge and will require retraining of all surgeons. However, ultimately, the ability to offer both open and percutaneous options for carotid disease increases the likelihood that an interventionalist will make the correct choice for each patient.

REFERENCES

1. American Heart Association: *Heart Disease and Stroke Statistics: 2003 Update.* Dallas, American Heart Association, 2002.
2. DeBakey MH: Carotid endarterectomy revisited. *J Endovasc Surg* 3:4, 1996.
3. Rutherford R: *Vascular Surgery*, ed 5, vol 2. Philadelphia, WB Saunders, 2000, p 1713.
4. Beneficial effect of carotid endarterectomy in symptomatic patients with high-grade carotid stenosis. North American Symptomatic Carotid Endarterectomy Trial Collaborators. *N Engl J Med* 325:445-453, 1991.
5. Executive Committee for the Asymptomatic Carotid Atherosclerosis Study: Endarterectomy for asymptomatic carotid artery stenosis. *JAMA* 273:1421-1428, 1995.
6. Morasch MD, Parker MA, Feinglass J, et al: Carotid endarterectomy: Characterization of recent increases in procedure rates. *J Vasc Surg* 31: 901-909, 2000.
7. Huber TS, Durance PW, Kazmers A, et al: Effect of the Asymptomatic Carotid Atherosclerosis Study on carotid endarterectomy in Veterans Affairs medical centers. *Arch Surg* 132:1134-1139, 1997.
8. Hallett JW Jr, Pietropaoli JA Jr, Ilstrup DM, et al: Comparison of North American Symptomatic Carotid Endarterectomy Trial and population-based outcomes for carotid endarterectomy. *J Vasc Surg* 27:845-851, 1998.
9. Mayo SW, Eldrup-Jorgensen J, Lucas FL, et al: Carotid endarterectomy after NASCET and ACAS: A statewide study. North American Symptomatic Carotid Endarterectomy Trial. Asymptomatic Carotid Artery Stenosis Study. *J Vasc Surg* 27:1017-1023, 1998.

10. Ruby ST, Robinson D, Lynch JT, et al: Outcome analysis of carotid end-arterectomy in Connecticut: The impact of volume and specialty. *Ann Vasc Surg* 10:22-26, 1996.
11. Matsen SL, Perler BA, Brown PM, et al: The distribution of carotid end-arterectomy procedures among surgeons and hospitals in New York State: Is regionalization of specialized vascular care occurring? *J Vasc Surg* 36:1146-1153, 2002.
12. Cebul RD, Snow RJ, Pine R, et al: Indications, outcomes, and provider volumes for carotid endarterectomy. *JAMA* 279:1282-1287, 1998.
13. Kresowik TF, Hemann RA, Grund SL, et al: Improving the outcomes of carotid endarterectomy: Results of a statewide quality improvement project. *J Vasc Surg* 31:918-926, 2000.
14. Reed AB, Gaccione P, Belkin M, et al: Preoperative risk factors for carotid endarterectomy: Defining the patient at high risk. *J Vasc Surg* 37:1191-1199, 2003.
15. Gasparis AP, Ricotta L, Cuadra SA, et al: High-risk carotid endarterectomy: Fact or fiction. *J Vasc Surg* 37:40-46, 2003.
16. Lepore MR Jr, Sternbergh WC III, Salartash K, et al: Influence of NASCET/ACAS trial eligibility on outcome after carotid endarterectomy. *J Vasc Surg* 34:581-586, 2001.
17. Jordan WD Jr, Alcocer F, Wirthlin DJ, et al: High-risk carotid endarterectomy: Challenges for carotid stent protocols. *J Vasc Surg* 35:16-21, 2002.
18. Illig KA, Zhang R, Tanski W, et al: Is the rationale for carotid angioplasty and stenting in patients excluded from NASCET/ACAS or eligible for ARCHeR justified? *J Vasc Surg* 37:575-581, 2003.
19. Bettmann MA, Katzen BT, Whisnant J, et al: Carotid stenting and angioplasty: A statement for healthcare professionals from the Councils on Cardiovascular Radiology, Stroke, Cardio-Thoracic and Vascular Surgery, Epidemiology and Prevention, and Clinical Cardiology, American Heart Association. *Stroke* 29:336-338, 1998.
20. Theron JG, Payelle GG, Coshun O, et al: Carotid artery stenosis: Treatment with protected balloon angioplasty and stent placement. *Radiology* 201:627-636, 1996.
21. Yadav JS, Roubin GS, Iyer SS, et al: Elective stenting of the extracranial carotid arteries. *Circulation* 95:376-381, 1997.
22. Wholey MH, Wholey MH, Tan WA, et al: A comparison of balloon-mounted and self-expanding stents in the carotid arteries: Immediate and long-term results of more than 500 patients. *J Endovasc Ther* 10:171-181, 2003
23. Dublin AB, Baltaxe HA, Cobb CA III. Percutaneous transluminal carotid angioplasty in fibromuscular dysplasia. Case report. *J Neurosurg* 59:162-165, 1983.
24. Bockenhimer SA, Mathias K: Percutaneous transluminal angioplasty in arteriosclerotic internal carotid artery stenosis. *Am J Neuroradiol* 4:791-792, 1983.

25. Wiggli U, Gratzl O: Transluminal angioplasty of stenotic carotid arteries: Case reports and protocol. *Am J Neuroradiol* 4:793-795, 1983.

26. Numaguchi Y, Puyau FA, Provenza LJ, et al: Percutaneous transluminal angioplasty of the carotid artery. Its application to post surgical stenosis. *Neuroradiology* 26:527-530, 1984.

27. Tsai FY, Matovich VB, Hieshima GB, et al: Practical aspects of percutaneous transluminal angioplasty of the carotid artery. *Acta Radiol Suppl* 369:127-130, 1986.

28. Endovascular versus surgical treatment in patients with carotid stenosis in the Carotid and Vertebral Artery Transluminal Angioplasty Study (CAVATAS): A randomised trial. *Lancet* 357:1729-1737, 2001.

29. Brooks WH, McClure RR, Jones MR, et al: Carotid angioplasty and stenting versus carotid endarterectomy: Randomized trial in a community hospital. *J Am Coll Cardiol* 38:1589-1595, 2001.

30. Yadav JS, for the SAPPHIRE investigators: Stenting and angioplasty with protection in patients at high risk for endarterectomy: The SAPPHIRE study. *Circulation* 106:2986A, 2003.

31. Wholey MH, Al-Mubarak N, Wholey MH: Updated review of the global carotid artery stent registry. *Cathet Cardiovasc Interv* 60:259-266, 2003.

32. Wholey MH, Wholey M, Mathias K, et al: Global experience in cervical carotid artery stent placement. *Cathet Cardiovasc Interv* 50:160-167, 2000.

33. Hobson RW II: CREST (Carotid Revascularization Endarterectomy versus Stent Trial): Background, design, and current status. *Semin Vasc Surg* 13:139-143, 2000.

34. Roubin GS: Dear editor-in-chief. *AJNR Am J Neuroradiol* 20:1378-1381, 1999.

35. Wholey MH, Jarmolowski CR, Wholey M, et al: Carotid artery stent placement: Ready for prime time? *J Vasc Interv Radiol* 14:1-10, 2003.

36. O'Donnell TF Jr, Rodriguez AA, Fortunato JE, et al: Management of recurrent carotid stenosis: Should asymptomatic lesions be treated surgically? *J Vasc Surg* 24:207-212, 1996.

37. Yadav JS, Roubin GS, King P, et al: Angioplasty and stenting for restenosis after carotid endarterectomy. Initial experience. *Stroke* 27:2075-2079, 1996.

38. New G, Roubin GS, Iyer SS, et al: Safety, efficacy, and durability of carotid artery stenting for restenosis following carotid endarterectomy: A multicenter study. *J Endovasc Ther* 7:345-352, 2000.

39. Alric P, Branchereau P, Berthet JP, et al: Carotid artery stenting for stenosis following revascularization or cervical irradiation. *J Endovasc Ther* 9:14-19, 2002.

40. Al-Mubarak N, Roubin GS, Iyer SS, et al: Carotid stenting for severe radiation-induced extracranial carotid artery occlusive disease. *J Endovasc Ther* 7:36-40, 2000.

41. Rockman CB, Jacobowitz GR, Adelman MA, et al: The benefits of carotid endarterectomy in the octogenarian: A challenge to the results of carotid angioplasty and stenting. *Ann Vasc Surg* 17:9-14, 2003.

42. Ahmadi R, Schillinger M, Lang W, et al: Carotid artery stenting in older patients: Is age a risk factor for poor outcome? *J Endovasc Ther* 9:559-565, 2002.

43. Wholey MH, Wholey MH, Eles G, et al: Evaluation of glycoprotein IIb /IIIa inhibitors in carotid angioplasty and stenting. *J Endovasc Ther* 10: 33-41, 2003.

44. Qureshi AI: Adjunctive use of platelet glycoprotein IIb/IIIa inhibitors for carotid angioplasty and stent placement: Time to say good bye? *J Endovasc Ther* 10:42-44, 2003.

45. Macdonald S, McKevitt F, Venables GS, et al: Neurological outcomes after carotid stenting protected with the NeuroShield filter compared to unprotected stenting. *J Endovasc Ther* 9:777-785, 2002.

46. Cremonesi A, Manetti R, Setacci F, et al: Protected carotid stenting: Clinical advantages and complications of embolic protection devices in 442 consecutive patients. *Stroke* 34:1936-1941, 2003.

47. Kastrup A, Groschel K, Krapf H, et al: Early outcome of carotid angioplasty and stenting with and without cerebral protection devices: A systematic review of the literature. *Stroke* 34:813-819, 2003.

48. Al-Mubarak N, Colombo A, Gaines PA, et al: Multicenter evaluation of carotid artery stenting with a filter protection system. *J Am Coll Cardiol* 39:841-846, 2002.

49. Castriota F, Cremonesi A, Manetti R, et al: Impact of cerebral protection devices on early outcome of carotid stenting. *J Endovasc Ther* 9:786-792, 2002.

50. Veith FJ, Amor M, Ohki T, et al: Current status of carotid bifurcation angioplasty and stenting based on a consensus of opinion leaders. *J Vasc Surg* 33:S111-S116, 2001.

51. Chang JB, Stein TA: Ten-year outcome after saphenous vein patch angioplasty in males and females after carotid endarterectomy. *J Vasc Endovasc Surg* 36:21-27, 2002.

52. Ballard JL, Romano M, Abou-Zamzam AM, et al: Carotid artery patch angioplasty: Impact and outcome. *Ann Vasc Surg* 16:12-16, 2002.

53. Cao P, DeRango P, Zannetti S: Eversion vs conventional carotid endarterectomy: A systematic review. *Eur J Vasc Endovasc Surg* 23:195-201. 2002.

54. Robbin ML, Lockhart ME, Weber TM, et al: Carotid artery stents: Early and intermediate follow-up with Doppler US. *Radiology* 205:749-756, 1997.

55. Christiaans MH, Ernst JM, Suttorp MJ, et al: Restenosis after carotid angioplasty and stenting: A follow-up study with duplex ultrasonography. *Eur J Vasc Endovasc Surg* 26:141-144, 2003.

56. Lal BK, Hobson RW, Goldstein J, et al: In-stent recurrent stenosis after carotid artery stenting: Life table analysis and clinical relevance. *J Vasc Surg* 38:1162-1168, 2003.

CHAPTER 4

Cerebral Protection Devices: What are the Options?

K. Kasirajan, MD

Assistant Professor of Surgery, Department of Surgery, Emory University School of Medicine, Atlanta, Ga

Carotid angioplasty is fast being incorporated into the treatment options for patients with carotid occlusive disease. The announcement of results of the SAPPHIRE and ARCHER trials have demonstrated that carotid angioplasty and stenting using cerebral protection devices is not inferior to open surgical endarterectomy.[1] The limiting step for percutaneous carotid interventions was the potential for cerebral embolization during the intervention.[2-4] The rapidly expanding field of embolic protection devices has offered an attractive array of devices that may be used for cerebral protection during carotid angioplasty and stenting.[5-7] This chapter reviews the various cerebral protection devices that are currently in clinical trials. The devices may be classified as flow occlusion devices, filters, and retrograde flow devices (Table 1).

FLOW OCCLUSION DEVICES

These devices use a standard 0.014-in guidewire with a distal occlusion balloon. Once the lesion is crossed with the balloon, the balloon is inflated and all the subsequent intervention (angioplasty /stenting) is performed with the balloon occluding flow to the brain. After completion of the angioplasty and stenting of the target lesion, any embolic debris is aspirated before balloon deflation. Disadvantages of this technique include the potential for embolization when crossing the lesion with the occlusion device. Additional risk of embolization may occur if the embolic particles along the edges of the

TABLE 1.

Classification of Emboli Protection Devices for
Possible Use During Carotid Angioplasty and
Stenting

System	Company
Occlusion Balloons	
GuardWire	Medtronic
TriActiv	Kensey Nash
Guardian	Abbott Laboratories
Filters	
Accunet	Guidant
Angioguard	Cordis
FilterWire EX	Boston Scientific
Interceptor	Medtronic
IntraGuard	Sultzer ITI (eV3)
NeuroShield	Abbott Laboratories
Sci-Pro	Scion Cardio-Vascular
Spider	eV3
TRAP NFS	Microvena (eV3)
Retrograde Flow Devices	
Mo.Ma	Invatac
PAES	ArteriA

balloon are not completely aspirated ("aspiration shadow"). Although complete flow occlusion is the closest to open surgical clamping of the internal carotid, once the distal balloon is inflated, the lesion cannot be further imaged until balloon deflation (Fig 1). Furthermore, not all patients will tolerate unilateral occlusion of the internal carotid artery for the time necessary to perform angioplasty and stenting. These disadvantages have resulted in a greater appeal for the embolic protection filters.

PERCUSURGE GUARDWIRE

The GuardWire Plus system (Medtronic, Santa Rosa, Calif) consists of 4 components, the first being a 0.014-in Teflon-coated guidewire (in lengths of 200 and 300 cm) constructed of hollow, kink-resistant nitinol hypotube in a helical design that provides for high flexibility and kink resistance. A low-pressure, highly compliant occlusion balloon is located at the proximal end of the distal tip of the wire. The distal tip of the wire is a radiopaque platinum coil similar to those found on standard guidewires. The current generation system features a crossing profile of 0.036 in. At its proximal end, the Guard-Wire incorporates the removable MicroSeal Adapter, which provides a means to open and close the internal MicroSeal (the inflation and deflation valve) in both rapid exchange and over-the-wire designs. Inflation is facilitated by the EZ Flator, a controlled volume syringe system that delivers diluted contrast fluid to inflate the balloon to between 3.0 and 6.0 mm in 0.5-mm increments by using a dial mechanism. The occlusion balloon remains inflated on detachment of the MicroSeal, after which the intervention is performed. To complete the procedure, the dual-lumen Export aspirating catheter is advanced over the GuardWire through its smaller lumen, and manual suction is applied to remove any collected emboli through the larger aspiration lumen before the balloon is deflated and the wire is withdrawn. A new-generation GuardWire device has been developed with a lower crossing profile of 0.028 in, which is currently available and has the added advantage that it can be passed through a standard 5F catheter.

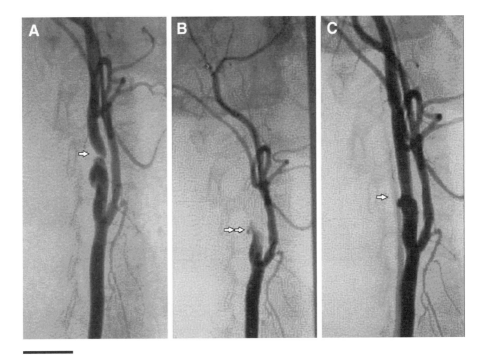

FIGURE 1.

A, High-grade carotid stenosis seen on a selective carotid angiogram. **B,** GuardWire occlusion demonstrates complete flow elimination. (Note difficulty in imaging target lesion during balloon protection.) **C,** Completion angiogram.

The GuardWire system is currently being evaluated in a number of randomized carotid stent studies, including Medtronic's PASCAL (Performance and Safety of the Medtronic AVE Self-Expandable Stent in Treatment of Carotid Artery Lesions) European carotid stent trial. The US clinical trial, known as MAVErIC (Evaluation of the Medtronic AVE Self-Expanding Carotid Stent System with Distal Protection in the Treatment of Carotid Stenosis), is a high-risk registry that has currently completed enrollment for its phase I study. The GuardWire was also part of the prospective nonrandomized CARESS (Carotid Artery Revascularization Endarterectomy versus Stenting Systems) trial that has completed enrollment for its feasibility phase of the study.

TRIACTIV

The TriActiv system (Kensey Nash Corp, Exton, Pa) consists of a stainless steel hypotube 0.014-in guidewire with a compliant, latex-based balloon mounted on its distal end. Currently, the guidewire length is 335 cm long. The distal balloon has a crossing profile of 0.034 in. Upon inflation with a prefilled carbon dioxide syringe, which allows for much more rapid inflation and deflation (averaging 1-2 seconds and 5 seconds, respectively) than contrast-based systems, the balloon expands to a diameter ranging from 3.0 to 5.0 mm. Inflation is accomplished at a low pressure of 2 atm, with lateral wall pressure well below 1 atm. Both the flush catheter (3F) and guidewire have radiopaque markers to enhance positioning under fluoroscopic visualization. The pole-mounted TriActiv system drive console features 6 preset operational modes, step-by-step on-screen instructions, and automated pumps for saline infusion and extraction. Fluid removal is accomplished at a rate of 150 mL of saline or blood per minute, whereas saline infusion occurs at 50 mL per minute. The latest generation is compatible with 8F guide catheters.

GUARDIAN

The Guardian (Abbott Laboratories/Rubicon Medical, Salt Lake City, Utah) is an occlusion balloon/aspiration catheter system that Rubicon is currently codeveloping with Abbott. Little information is currently available on this device, as it remains in its preclinical test stage.

DISTAL FILTER DEVICES

Distal embolic protection filters often consist of a delivery catheter, a filter guidewire, and a separate retrieval catheter. The filter guidewires comprise a distally mounted filter, which is advanced through

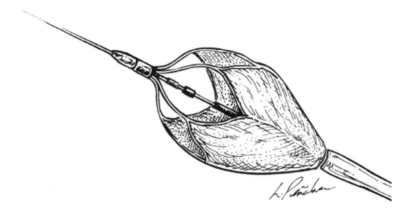

FIGURE 2.
AccuNet. (Courtesy of Kasirajan K, Schneider PA, Kent KC: Emboli protection filters for cerebral protection during carotid angioplasty and stenting. *J Endovasc Ther* 10:21-27, 2003. Reprinted with permission.)

the delivery catheter for crossing the stenosis, before angioplasty and stent placement. A metal with thermal memory, such as nitinol, is often used in the construction of either the filter itself or the filter frame structure, allowing for the collapse of the element within the delivery and retrieval catheter. Once the device is maneuvered beyond the stenosis, retraction of the delivery catheter opens the filter, which then traps released debris during the angioplasty. After the protected procedure is completed, the retrieval catheter is advanced, completely enveloping the filtration element, and then the entire device along with any trapped emboli is removed. Pores within the filter permit distal blood flow, which allows the use of contrast imaging for continued intraoperative visualization in addition to reducing the risk of ischemic events. Disadvantages include the risk of embolization when crossing the target lesion with the filter. Filter thrombosis and clogging with embolic debris, although rare, may eliminate the advantage of a filter over an occlusion device.

ACCUNET
The AccuNet system (Guidant, Indianapolis, Ind) comprises a polyurethane filter over a nitinol basket. The basket expands to diameters ranging from 4 to 8 mm, and the filter pore size is 120 μm or less (Fig 2). The AccuNet is based on Guidant's ACE Hi-Torque Balance Heavyweight guidewire with a 0.014-in diameter and a 300-cm length. The results of the ARCHER (Acculink for Revascularization

of Carotids in High Risk Patients) trial for high-risk patients were recently announced at the American College of Cardiology in March 2003. Technical success was achieved in 92.7% of patients, and visible embolic debris was seen in 57% of the baskets retrieved. Overall, the stroke rate was 5.3%, death rate was 2.3%, and myocardial infarction rate was 2.1%. The major ipsilateral stroke rate was 1.4%.

ANGIOGUARD

The AngioGuard Emboli Capture Guidewire system (Cordis Endovascular, Warren, NJ) consists of a standard 0.014-in guidewire with an expandable nitinol basket filter attached to its distal end. Upon retraction of the delivery sheath, the basket expands up to 8 mm and is collapsible for device removal. The filter has multiple 100-µm laser-drilled holes that permit perfusion (Fig 3). The current generation AngioGuard XP features a reduced profile for improved crossability. The corresponding basket sizes and crossing profiles are 4 mm (3.2F), 5 mm (3.3F), 6 mm (3.5F), 7 mm (3.7F), and 8 mm (4.0F).

The SAPPHIRE (Study of Angioplasty with Protection in Patients at High Risk for Endarterectomy) trial has completed enrollment, and 1-month and 1-year data have been announced (Table 2). This is the first prospective study comparing standard carotid endarterectomy (CEA) with carotid angioplasty and stenting (CAS) using an emboli protection device. The composite end point of death, stroke, and myocardial infarction was statistically in favor of CAS (CAS 5.8%, CEA 12.6%; P = .047). Interestingly, the major ipsilateral stroke rate for CAS was 0% and 1.3% for CEA.

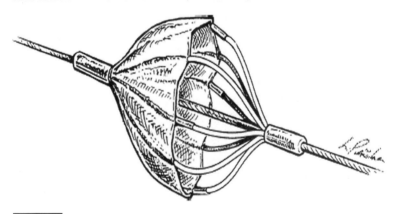

FIGURE 3.

AngioGuard. (Courtesy of Kasirajan K, Schneider PA, Kent KC: Emboli protection filters for cerebral protection during carotid angioplasty and stenting. *J Endovasc Ther* 10:21-27, 2003. Reprinted with permission.)

TABLE 2.
Results of the SAPPHIRE Carotid Angioplasty Versus Endarterectomy Trial

Primary End Points	CAS	CEA	P Value
Number	156	151	
Death	0.6%	2%	.36
Stroke	3.8%	5.3%	.59
MI	2.6%	7.3%	.07

Abbreviations: *CAS*, Carotid angioplasty and stenting; *CEA*, carotid endarterectomy; *MI*, myocardial infarction.

FILTERWIRE EX

The FilterWire (Boston Scientific, Maple Grove, Minn) consists of an expandable nitinol loop structure mounted off-center on a standard 0.014-in guidewire, used with a 2.9F delivery/retrieval sheath. A thin polyurethane filter with 80-µm pores is attached to the loop structure and rotates freely on the end of the guidewire. The nitinol loop facilitates fluoroscopic visualization and features an open, or "fish" mouth, which acts as the filter basket and retains the trapped emboli during retrieval (Fig 4). The expandable nature of the elliptical loop permits the treatment of vessels between 3.0 and 5.5 mm with a single device. Two trials are currently underway: the CABERNET (Carotid Artery Revascularization Using the Boston Scientific EPI FilterWire EX and the EndoTex NexStent) study, which will en-

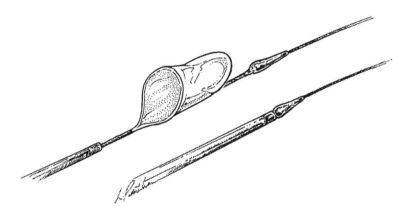

FIGURE 4.
FilterWire. (Courtesy of Kasirajan K, Schneider PA, Kent KC: Emboli protection filters for cerebral protection during carotid angioplasty and stenting. *J Endovasc Ther* 10:21-27, 2003. Reprinted with permission.)

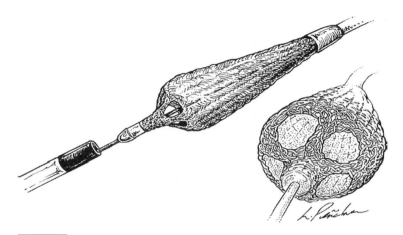

FIGURE 5.

Interceptor. (Courtesy of Kasirajan K, Schneider PA, Kent KC: Emboli protection filters for cerebral protection during carotid angioplasty and stenting. *J Endovasc Ther* 10:21-27, 2003. Reprinted with permission.)

roll patients (n = 600) at high risk for CEA in 30 US and European centers; and the Boston Scientific/EPI (BEACH) clinical trial (n = 776), which will evaluate the magic wall stent (Boston Scientific) with the FilterWire for distal protection.

INTERCEPTOR

The Interceptor (Medtronic, Santa Rosa, Calif) is a 7F-compatible, low-profile, flexible, self-expanding, braided nitinol filter that has 4 large proximal entry ports and a tapered proximal surface to facilitate the entrance of emboli, while 110-μm distal pores permit perfusion (Fig 5). The system is based on a standard 0.014-in wire platform with delivery and retrieval sheath diameters of 4.2F and 4.5F, respectively. No carotid trials are currently underway.

INTRAGUARD

Based on a 0.014-in guidewire, the 4F IntraGuard (Sulzer Intra-Therapeutics [Centerpulse]/eV3, Plymouth, Minn) is designed to treat vessels ranging in size from 3 to 7 mm (Fig 6). The system features a nitinol frame with a patented, retractable "flower petal" design that supports a synthetic microfilter with 100-μm pores. Currently, Sulzer IntraTherapeutics has been acquired by eV3. Since eV3 has its own emboli protection device (Spider), further development and trials with the Intraguard are questionable.

NEUROSHIELD

The Neuroshield (Abbott Laboratories/MedNova, Abbott Park, Ill) consists of a delivery catheter, a filter delivery wire, a support wire (featuring a nitinol filtration element mounted on its distal tip), and a retrieval catheter. The filtration element, which has large entry ports at the proximal end and multiple 140-µm perfusion pores at the distal end, contains a preshaped nitinol expansion system. Radiopaque marker bands are located at the proximal and distal ends of the 2.5-mm-long filtration element to enhance visualization. The guidewire is 315 cm long with a usable length of 135 cm. The current device features a bare wire configuration that permits lesion crossing with an independent filter delivery wire (a 0.014-in polytetrafluoroethylene [PTFE]-coated guidewire that tapers to 0.018 in at its distal end). A range of support wires is offered with filtration elements available in diameters of 4.0, 5.0, and 6.0 mm to permit the treatment of vessels ranging in size from 3.5 to 6.2 mm (Fig 7). Crossing profiles for the delivery and retrieval catheters are 3.0F and 6.5F, respectively. A recent multicenter European study evaluated the NeuroShield in 162 patients undergoing carotid artery stenting. Of the 164 hemispheres treated, angiographic success was achieved in 162 (99%), with successful filter placement in 154 (94%). Of the 10 unsuccessful cases, carotid access could not be attained in 2 (1%), and filters could not be placed in 8 (5%). Five procedures were performed with no embolic protection, whereas protection for the other 3 procedures was established with other devices. The overall 30-day

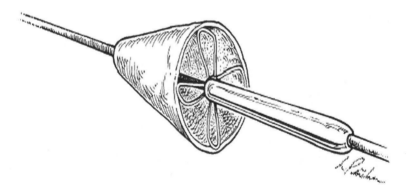

FIGURE 6.

IntraGuard. (Courtesy of Kasirajan K, Schneider PA, Kent KC: Emboli protection filters for cerebral protection during carotid angioplasty and stenting. *J Endovasc Ther* 10:21-27, 2003. Reprinted with permission.)

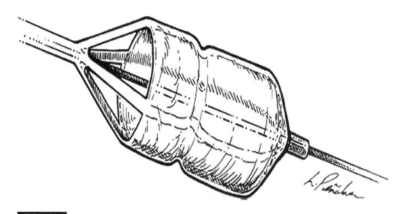

FIGURE 7.

NeuroShield. (Courtesy of Kasirajan K, Schneider PA, Kent KC: Emboli protection filters for cerebral protection during carotid angioplasty and stenting. *J Endovasc Ther* 10:21-27, 2003. Reprinted with permission.)

event rate of 2% included 4 total events: 2 minor strokes (one of which occurred in a patient without protection) and 2 deaths (one from cardiac arrhythmia and one from hyperperfusion-related intracerebral hemorrhage). There were no major embolic strokes.[8] In the United States, the NeuroShield is currently being evaluated by the SECURITY trial (a Registry Study to Evaluate the NeuroShield Bare Wire Cerebral Protection System and X.act Stent in Patients at High Risk for Carotid Endarterectomy).

SCI-PRO

The Sci-Pro (Scion Cardio-Vascular, Miami, Fla) consists of a guidewire and basket filter, as with other distal filter systems. However, while most other systems involve the pullback of a delivery sheath/catheter to deploy the filter (and the subsequent advancement of a retrieval catheter to collapse the filter), the basket of the Sci-Pro is activated through an inner core wire by mechanical means. Simply pushing or pulling the proximal wire expands or collapses the basket filter, respectively. The device is available in multiple configurations, including proximal guidewire diameters of 0.014, 0.018, and 0.035 in and wire lengths between 150 and 300 cm. The inner core wire is made of 304 stainless steel, and the baskets, available in diameters ranging from 4 to 7 mm, are made of nitinol. The filter itself consists of a polyurethane membrane with 190-μm holes attached to the distal half of the basket (Fig 8). The Sci-Pro system is compatible with 6F guiding catheters.

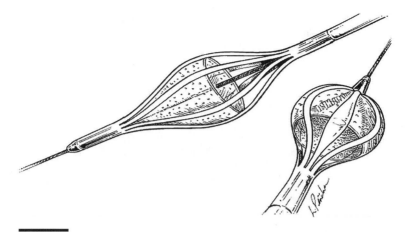

FIGURE 8.

Sci-Pro. (Courtesy of Kasirajan K, Schneider PA, Kent KC: Emboli protection filters for cerebral protection during carotid angioplasty and stenting. *J Endovasc Ther* 10:21-27, 2003. Reprinted with permission.)

SPIDER

The Spider (eV3, Plymouth, Minn) has a unique nitinol filter design that is capable of trapping particles as small as 36 µm (Fig 9). This is currently the smallest pore size of any available embolic protection filter system. A radiopaque proximal gold loop helps in complete circumferential vessel apposition for complete capture of embolic debris. It has a 2.9F crossing profile and is 6F guide catheter com-

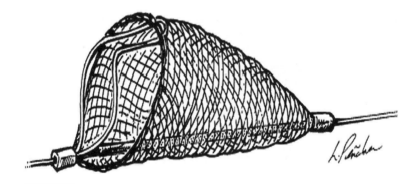

FIGURE 9.

Spider. (Courtesy of Kasirajan K, Schneider PA, Kent KC: Emboli protection filters for cerebral protection during carotid angioplasty and stenting. *J Endovasc Ther* 10:21-27, 2003. Reprinted with permission.)

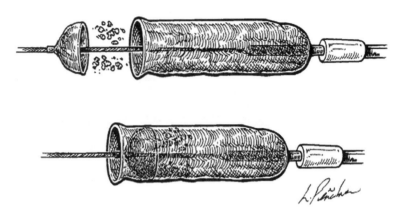

FIGURE 10.

TRAP-NFS. (Courtesy of Kasirajan K, Schneider PA, Kent KC: Emboli protection filters for cerebral protection during carotid angioplasty and stenting. *J Endovasc Ther* 10:21-27, 2003. Reprinted with permission.)

patible, and heparin coating of the filter basket is provided to prevent thrombosis during prolonged and complex interventions. It is manufactured in diameters of 3.0, 4.0, 5.0, 6.0, and 7.0 mm, with a usable guidewire length of 320 cm. The Spider also has a unique snap wire feature to convert to a 175-cm rapid exchange configuration.

TRAP NFS

Microvena Corporation/eV3 (Plymouth, Minn) has developed the TRAP neurofilter system (NFS) designed for carotid application. The devices consist of a nitinol-braided mesh basket, featuring a heparin coating to reduce the risk of thrombosis, mounted on a PTFE-coated stainless steel guidewire, in addition to the 3.5F delivery and 5F to 6F recovery catheters (Fig 10). Basket diameters of 2.5, 3.0, 3.5, 4.0, 5.0, 6.0, and 7.0 mm are available. The potential for embolization of the captured particulate matter during recapture of the filter basket is minimized by retracting the distal basket into a proximal nitinol mesh basket.

RETROGRADE FLOW DEVICES

Proximal balloon occlusion represents yet another method of embolic protection that addresses one of the major shortcomings of distal protection devices: unprotected lesion crossing. Distal filters and distal balloon occlusion devices require guidewire crossing of the lesion before protection is in place, but proximal balloon occlusion devices establish protection beforehand, which may potentially lead to improved clinical results. The main disadvantage is the large profile of these devices that significantly reduces their trackability across difficult aortic arches. In addition, up to 10% of patients may not tolerate a "cerebral steal" resulting from the retrograde flow of blood away from the brain.

PARODI ANTI-EMBOLI SYSTEM

The Parodi Anti-Emboli System (PAES; ArteriA Medical Science, San Francisco, Calif) consists of the 8F inner diameter Parodi Anti-Emboli Catheter (PAEC), the low-profile Parodi External Balloon (PEB), and the Parodi Blood Return Set (PBRS), an arterial-venous shunt with a 180-µm perfusion filter. The PAEC is a guiding catheter with a funnel-shaped occlusion balloon at its distal tip. The PAEC is inserted through the femoral artery and placed in the common carotid artery, where its occlusion balloon is inflated, maintaining access to the lesion through its main lumen. The PEB is inserted through the main lumen of the PAEC and inflated in the external carotid artery to prevent retrograde flow from the external back into the internal carotid artery. With the high-pressure internal carotid artery now isolated, the PBRS is attached to an outlet port at the proximal end of the PAEC catheter and inserted through an introducer sheath into the low-pressure femoral vein. The high-pressure to low-pressure connection induces natural and passive continuous flow reversal down the internal carotid artery (Fig 11). Embolic debris then flows through the PAEC and is captured by the filter in the PBRS before blood is returned to the femoral vein. In cases done with transcranial Doppler monitoring, physicians have observed 0 HITS (high-intensity signals, representing embolic particles, including air) traveling to the brain. In addition to establishing complete protection before any interaction with the lesion, the PAES is capable of capturing emboli of all sizes and permits physicians to use their guidewire of choice. Limitations of the PAES include flow interruption and a larger femoral puncture site because of the current 10F size of the system.

MO.MA

The Mo.Ma (Invatec, France) is based on the concept of interrupting blood flow in the zone of the carotid bifurcation through the use of 2 occlusion balloons: one for the common carotid artery and the other for the external carotid artery, similar to ArteriA's PAES. Unlike the PAES, the Mo.Ma accomplishes occlusion of both arteries with a single device that is capable of adapting itself to carotids of varying

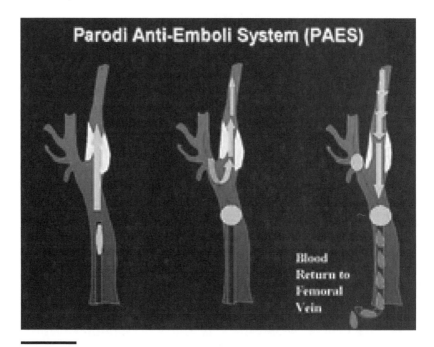

FIGURE 11.
Parodi Anti-Emboli System (PAES). (Courtesy of Parodi JC, Schonholz C, Ferreira LM, et al: "Seat belt and air bag" technique for cerebral protection during carotid stenting. *J Endovasc Ther* 9:20-24, 2002. Reprinted with permssion.)

diameters via extremely compliant balloons, and embolic debris (along with blood) is aspirated out of the body. The Mo.Ma catheter consists of a number of segments of varying stiffness for optimized tracking and delivery.

CONCLUSION

The rapid development and improvement in the science of emboli protection systems may help hasten the introduction of CAS as an acceptable alternative to open surgical revascularization. The availability of various devices for distal protection may also help physicians tailor devices specific for each patient's anatomy. The future of carotid interventions will probably be driven by patients' demand for less invasive procedures with shorter recovery times.

REFERENCES

1. Yadav J TSI: Stenting and Angioplasty with Protection in Patients at High Risk for Endarterectomy: The Sapphire Study. *Circulation* 106: 2002.

2. Cohen JE, Lylyk P, Ferrario A, et al: Carotid stent angioplasty: The role of cerebral protection devices. *Neurol Res* 25:162-168, 2003.

3. Grube E, Colombo A, Hauptmann E, et al: Initial multicenter experience with a novel distal protection filter during carotid artery stent implantation. *Cathet Cardiovasc Interv* 58:139-146, 2003.

4. Hobson RW II, Lal BK, Chaktoura E, et al: Carotid artery stenting: Analysis of data for 105 patients at high risk. *J Vasc Surg* 37:1234-1239, 2003.

5. Kastrup A, Groschel K, Krapf H, et al: Early outcome of carotid angioplasty and stenting with and without cerebral protection devices: A systematic review of the literature. *Stroke* 34:813-819, 2003.

6. Wholey MH, Tan WA, Eles G, et al: Comparison of balloon-mounted and self-expanding stents in the carotid arteries: Immediate and long-term results of more than 500 patients. *J Endovasc Ther* 10:171-181, 2003.

7. Wholey MH, Wholey M: Current status in cervical carotid artery stent placement. *J Cardiovasc Surg (Torino)* 44:331-339, 2003.

8. Al-Mubarak N, Colombo A, Gaines PA, et al: Multicenter evaluation of carotid artery stenting with a filter protection system. *J Am Coll Cardiol* 39:841-846, 2002.

CHAPTER 5

Devices for Endovascular Abdominal Aortic Aneurysm Repair: Factors Affecting Stent Graft Selection

Peter L. Faries, MD, FACS

Chief of Endovascular Surgery, Division of Vascular Surgery, New York-Presbyterian Hospital, Cornell University, Weill Medical College, Columbia University, College of Physicians and Surgeons, New York, NY

ABSTRACT

Minimally invasive endovascular techniques for the treatment of abdominal aortic aneurysms (AAA) have significantly reduced the morbidity of these procedures as compared with standard surgical repair. In addition, patients with extensive comorbid medical illnesses in whom standard operative repair is contraindicated may be successfully treated using endovascular means. A variety of endovascular stent grafts are currently being used clinically for endovascular AAA repair. The characteristics of these stent grafts vary significantly. In selecting the specific stent graft to be used for endovascular AAA repair, these specific characteristics must be considered, particularly with regard to the individual patient's anatomic and physiologic characteristics. In addition, the indications for use of endovascular grafts as compared with standard open surgery have not yet been fully defined. Endovascular stent grafts in current use have limitations, and their use must be tempered accordingly until their long-term effectiveness is more completely evaluated. This chapter describes the general principles of use for endovascular devices for the repair of AAAs. It details the features and results for the devices in current use and highlights the factors that influence the selection of specific stent-graft types.

R epair of abdominal aortic aneurysms (AAAs) is performed to prevent progressive expansion and rupture. AAA rupture results in considerable morbidity and mortality as well as significant cost to society.[1] The rate of occurrence of AAAs has been estimated to be 60 per 1000 in the general population by epidemiologic studies,[2] and an incidence between 1.8% and 6.6% has been observed in autopsy studies.[1,3] The natural history of AAAs was studied in patients before the advent of surgical repair and in patients who have been unable to undergo AAA repair. In these studies, the rate of aneurysm rupture and death could exceed 60% within 3 years of the initial diagnosis.[4] Surgical repair was first reported in 1962 and remains the only effective treatment of AAAs.[5] Mortality rates ranging from 3% to 5% have been reported for elective standard operative repair of uncomplicated cases in major vascular centers.[6] However, these rates increase significantly in patients with significant comorbid medical conditions, particularly coronary artery disease, renal failure, and chronic obstructive pulmonary disease.

Federal estimates indicate that more than 15,000 deaths caused by aneurysm rupture occur each year in the United States.[7] At least 62% of patients who experience rupture of an AAA have been estimated to die before reaching the hospital.[8] When in-hospital deaths are included, the overall mortality rate for ruptured AAAs is thought to approach 90%.[8-10] In addition to the significant loss of life associated with AAA rupture, there are considerable health care costs. Cost reimbursement studies document an average loss to the hospital of approximately $25,000 per patient presenting with a ruptured AAA.[11] It is estimated that 2000 lives and $50 million could be saved annually in the United States alone if aortic aneurysms were repaired before rupture.[12]

CURRENT INDICATIONS FOR ENDOVASCULAR REPAIR

As experience with the use of stent grafts has increased, the indications and the anatomic selection criteria for endovascular repair of AAAs have evolved. Conclusive agreement on what these indications should be has not yet been reached. During the initial experience with endovascular AAA repair, patients were offered endovascular treatment on a compassionate-need basis. Endovascular grafts were used to treat patients who had aneurysms that were at significant risk for rupture, but who could not tolerate standard surgical repair. Endovascular repair remains the most appropriate treatment choice for these patients. However, the use of endovascular devices to treat AAAs in patients who would be candidates for open surgical repair has significantly increased. Recent studies have indicated lower perioperative morbidity and mortality rates for patients undergoing endovascular as compared with conventional AAA repair. The decision to use endovascular techniques to treat AAAs is also influenced by the anatomic constraints of the endovascular device.

ANATOMIC SELECTION CRITERIA

A number of anatomic and technical criteria must be fulfilled to enable endovascular repair of AAAs to be performed successfully. These criteria include:

1. The presence of an undilated segment of aorta distal to the renal ostia that is of sufficient length to allow implantation of the proximal aspect of the endovascular device; this is the proximal neck. The length of normal proximal aorta necessary for device implantation varies according to the specifications of the individual device. The recommended length ranges from 1.0 to 1.5 cm.
2. Severe angulation of the proximal neck may also preclude endovascular treatment. In general, treatment of aneurysms with an angle less than 60º between the suprarenal aorta and the proximal neck is not recommended by the manufacturers, although variation according to the specific device type ultimately determines the maximum acceptable angle.
3. If the site selected for distal implantation is the iliac artery, its morphology must be adequate for seating of the distal attachment system of the endovascular device.
4. The common and external iliac arteries must be of sufficient caliber to allow passage of the introducer sheath, or must be amenable to balloon dilatation to facilitate passage.
5. The iliac vessels must demonstrate limited tortuosity to enable the delivery system for the stent graft to be advanced into the aorta. Variation in the flexibility and trackability of delivery systems for stent-graft deployment may affect their utilization in tortuous iliac vessels.
6. Aberrant vessels, particularly an indispensable inferior mesenteric or accessory renal artery, must not be present in the segment of aorta to be excluded from the circulation.

If these criteria are not met, it may not be possible to carry out the procedures because of technical reasons.

PREOPERATIVE ASSESSMENT

Radiologic assessment of the AAA and iliac vessels is performed to determine the diameter and length of the endovascular device to be used. A screening computed tomographic (CT) scan with intravenous contrast is most commonly performed. Ideally, a high-speed helical scanner is used to obtain images at 3-mm intervals. Three-dimensional reconstruction images may also be obtained. The dimensions of the proximal and distal aortic necks as well as the aneurysm length and composition may be calculated from these studies. In addition, the length of the endovascular graft necessary for treatment of the aneurysm may be estimated with 3-dimensional reconstruction of the CT. Angiography with a calibrated catheter with radiopaque markers at 1-cm intervals may also be used in the assessment of arterial length and to assess adjacent arterial structures. This catheter allows for the compensation of parallax and magnification, permitting accurate determination of the length of graft necessary for endovascular treatment.[13]

DEPLOYMENT OF ENDOVASCULAR DEVICES

Endovascular AAA repair is most commonly performed in the operating room. This environment is the safest and the best suited to handle potential complications that might be encountered, including iliac artery perforation, damage to the femoral access site, aortic thrombosis, and the need to rapidly convert to an open repair. Also, since these procedures involve the introduction of a vascular graft, sterile technique is of the utmost importance; some investigators believe that this is best maintained in the operating room.[13]

Before surgery, the patient is fully prepared and draped in a sterile manner. The endovascular procedure is performed under fluoroscopic guidance. The operating room should be equipped with advanced fluoroscopic instruments and a radiolucent operating table. A radiopaque marked backboard or ruler may be placed beneath the patient to provide fluoroscopic reference measurements. Access to the arterial system is obtained either through exposure of the common femoral artery or, if this vessel is of inadequate caliber, through a limited retroperitoneal approach to the iliac artery. Once arterial access has been obtained, wire and catheter techniques are used to deploy the device. Considerable variation in deployment techniques exists between device types. These will frequently influence graft selection and are described subsequently.

After deployment of the endovascular graft, a completion arteriogram is performed. Some centers advocate the use of intravascular ultrasound to assess graft deployment and determine the presence of graft stenosis or kinking. Luminal narrowing, particularly in the iliac limbs of the graft, may be treated by balloon angioplasty. Stent placement may also be necessary to provide further support. Follow-up protocols vary, but typically include serial plane radiographs and abdominal CT scans, and may include color-flow duplex scanning or magnetic resonance imaging. If an abnormality or change from baseline is detected, arteriography may be performed to fully evaluate the status of the graft and the implantation sites as well as any persistent perfusion of the aneurysm sac.

COMMERCIALLY FABRICATED ENDOVASCULAR DEVICES

After the initial success of endovascular stent grafts fabricated by vascular surgeons, commercially manufactured endovascular devices were developed. These devices have received considerable clinical exposure and have entered into widespread use. Three have received approval from the US Food and Drug Administration (FDA): (1) AneuRx (Medtronic, Inc, Minneapolis, Minn); (2) Excluder (W.L. Gore and Associates, Flagstaff, Ariz); and (3) Zenith (Cook, Inc, Bloomington, Ind). Five additional devices have received approval for use in the European Union or are in use in pivotal trials in the United States: (4) Talent (Medtronic); (5) Quantum (Cordis, Inc, Sommerville, NJ); (6) PowerLink (Endologix, Irvine, Calif); (7) LifePath (Baxter Healthcare Corp, Irvine, Calif); and (8) Anaconda (Sulzer Vascutek, Austin, Tex). One commercial device, the Ancure (Guidant Corp, Menlo Park, Calif), has been withdrawn from use.

ANEURX STENT-GRAFT SYSTEM

A modular, bifurcated, self-expanding stent-graft system has been developed by Medtronic. The modular components consist of a thin-walled, noncrimped, woven polyester graft supported by a nitinol (nickel-titanium alloy) frame along its entire length. Modular aortic and iliac extenders may also be added. All components are contained in delivery sheaths, which are introduced bilaterally through the femoral vessels. The AneuRx delivery system has recently been modified to facilitate placement without requirement of a sheath. The new delivery system uses a tapered tip and possesses considerably greater flexibility than the original system. In addition, the runners, which allow unsheathing of the device and which must be withdrawn after expansion of the stent graft, are now coated with Teflon to minimize friction and the chance of dislodging the stent graft from its desired position. The delivery system has an outer diameter size of 21F for the main aortic body of the graft and 16F for the contralateral modular iliac limb. The AneuRx stent graft may be used to treat proximal aortic neck diameters from 16 to 26 mm. Iliac limbs may be used to treat diameters up to 16 mm; however, use of an aortic extension cuff at the iliac implantation site has been described for the treatment of iliac diameters up to 24 mm.[14]

The results of a nonrandomized, multicenter clinical trial comparing endovascular AAA treatment with the AneuRx device with conventional open repair led to the original market approval from the US FDA.[15] In that study during an 18-month period, 190 patients underwent AAA repair with this device. The operative mortality rate was 2.6%. The overall morbidity rate was 17%, with a 12% major morbid event rate. These included myocardial infarction, stroke, renal failure, and arrhythmia. Minor morbidities, which occurred in 5% of the patients, included wound infection, minor toe embolization, mild femoral neuropathy, and an increase in creatinine level that did not require treatment. The use of the AneuRx device when compared with surgical treatment was found to offer advantages in reducing the rate of major morbidity and length of hospital stay.

In the 6-year follow-up of patients treated with the AneuRx stent graft, the device was found to have an implant success rate of 98% with a perioperative mortality rate of 1.9% (Table 1). Overall 1-year survival was 94%, and 4-year survival was 62.4%. Conversion to conventional repair was required in 4.4% during the 6-year follow-up, with AAA rupture occurring in 1.3% and being largely attributable to persistent endoleaks. The incidence of endoleak was 21% at 1 year and declined to 13% at 6 years.[16] Continuing follow-up of these patients remains ongoing.

GORE EXCLUDER ENDOPROSTHESIS

The Excluder stent-graft system is composed of thin-walled polytetrafluoroethylene (PTFE) externally supported throughout its length

---

TABLE 1.
Results of Medtronic AneuRx

Implant success	98%
30-Day mortality	1.9%
Perioperative conversion to standard open repair	1.3%
Conversion to conventional repair (at 4 years)	2.8%
Secondary procedures	8%
1-Year survival	94%
3-Year survival	84%
AAA rupture	0.8%%
Endoleak at 1 year	21%
Endoleak at 3 years	18%

Abbreviation: AAA, Abdominal aortic aneurysm.

TABLE 2.
Results of Gore Excluder

Implant success	100%
30-Day mortality	1%
Perioperative conversion to standard open repair	0%
Conversion to conventional repair (at 4 years)	1.5%
Secondary procedures	7%/y
Aortic component migration	1%
Iliac limb migration	1%
Endoleak at 1 year	17%
Endoleak at 2 years	20%

with nitinol stents. It is a modular bifurcated system. The main body is delivered through an 18F sheath, while the contralateral limb is delivered through a 12F sheath. There are no suture holes in the graft material; thus, the risk for leakage through fabric tears is reduced. There is an external sealing cuff at the proximal end to aid in fixation to the proximal attachment point. A PTFE fiber deployment line is pulled to permit rapid deployment of the device when it is positioned at the appropriate implantation site. The release occurs rapidly and without lengthening or shortening of the prosthesis. Incremental release is not possible, and the prosthesis may not be repositioned once released.

The pivotal trial has been completed for the Excluder. It has received approval from the US FDA and is currently being marketed. The results of the pivotal trial were recently reported.[17] A total of 528 patients were enrolled in the trial. The endoprosthesis was deployed successfully in all patients without the need for conversion to conventional aneurysm repair in any case (Table 2). Delayed conversion was required in 1.5% during the 2-year follow-up period. Conversion was performed most commonly for persistent endoleak and aneurysm expansion. Increase in aneurysm size after endovascular repair was seen in 14%, whereas aneurysm size reduction was documented in 19%. The overall need for aneurysm reintervention was 7% per year. When compared with the control patients in the trial who had undergone conventional aneurysm repair, the patients treated with the Excluder stent graft experienced significantly fewer major adverse events.

COOK ZENITH AAA ENDOVASCULAR GRAFT

The Zenith system from Cook is a modular bifurcated device that is also available in an aortouni-iliac configuration. It consists of woven polyester graft material supported throughout its length by self-expanding Z-stents. The introducer tip is tapered to minimize trauma at the arterial insertion site, and there are side holes at the tip to allow angiography with the system in place. The Zenith stent-graft system has a bare proximal stent that expands radially on deployment. There are barbs incorporated into the bare stent to secure the device to the suprarenal aortic wall. The suprarenal bare stent is deployed after being released by a trigger wire, which holds it in place to avoid premature deployment. The main aortic body is deployed with an 18F or 20F delivery system. The iliac limb is delivered using a 14F system. The Zenith device can be used in aortic necks up to 31 mm and in iliac arteries up to 22 mm. The system is designed to allow all components to be used together, and as a result, a greater range of anatomic sizes can be managed with the Zenith graft.

The midterm results for the use of the Cook Zenith graft have been published.[18] The device was used in 528 patients starting in 1995. The design of the device has evolved to its current form during the intervening years. The success rate for implantation was 99.3% (Table 3). Endoleaks have been observed in 15% in the perioperative period and decreased to 4% at 4 years, with an average follow-up of 14 months. Conversion to conventional repair was required in 4 patients, and device migration was seen in 8, although no migration has occurred with the current graft design. Late rupture occurred in 3 patients and was associated with endoleak. Based on the results of the pivotal trial, the Cook Zenith device has received approval for use in the United States from the FDA.

MEDTRONIC TALENT DEVICE

The endovascular stent graft developed by World Medical and Medtronic has been implanted in more than 18,000 patients world-

TABLE 3.
Results of Cook Zenith

Implant success	99.3%
Perioperative conversion to standard open repair	0.8%
Device migration	1.4%
Reduction in AAA diameter	58%
AAA diameter unchanged	33%
Endoleak at 30 days	15%
Endoleak at 4 years	4%
Late aneurysm rupture	0.6%

Abbreviation: AAA, Abdominal aortic aneurysm.

wide. The Talent graft is used in 2 configurations: tapered/aortouni-iliac and bifurcated/aortobi-iliac. It is self-expanding and composed of a Dacron graft with a nitinol frame that supports the graft. The proximal aortic fixation device possesses 1.5 cm of uncovered nitinol frame proximal to the fabric portion of the device. This uncovered portion permits transrenal fixation of the device, thereby allowing the treatment of AAAs with relatively short or angulated proximal necks. The graft may be custom fabricated for each patient individually and consequently can be used to treat a great range of aortic and iliac anatomic configurations. The Talent device may be used for proximal aortic neck sizes up to 34 mm and for iliac implantation site diameters up to 24 mm. Deployment of the device is similar to that of the AneuRx device, although runners are not required for delivery of the Talent device. The main aortic component with the ipsilateral iliac limb is delivered through a 22F or 24F system. The second contralateral iliac limb module is then deployed via the contralateral femoral artery with an 18F delivery sheath.

A recent report has been prepared summarizing the results of an FDA-sponsored investigational device exemption trial for high-risk patients.[19] In the US trial, all patients either had significant comorbid medical conditions or possessed a hostile abdomen. Technical success was achieved in 93% of patients treated with the Talent device. Secondary procedures were required in 8.7%. Conversion to open surgical repair was required in 1% of the cases. The overall 30-day mortality rate was 1.9%. From the reported experience, it was concluded that the Talent endovascular device was suitable for the treatment of AAAs in a significant proportion of medically high-risk patients.

CORDIS QUANTUM ENDOVASCULAR DEVICE

The Quantum device uses transrenal fixation of the proximal aspect of the endovascular graft, which appears to offer potential advantages in patients with short or angulated proximal necks. In addition, the Quantum graft incorporates the ability to adjust iliac graft length once an endovascular device has been inserted into the arterial system. This is necessary to provide maximal aneurysm exclusion. The Quantum endovascular aortic graft is constructed from seamless nitinol hypo-tube stents, which provide the thermal memory properties of the nitinol metal material. The attachment system is equipped with a transrenal segment, which optimizes renal artery blood flow while enhancing suprarenal fixation. Fully integrated self-deploying barbs engage the aortic wall immediately below the lowest renal artery. This region of the aorta has proven to be least susceptible to progressive dilatation as first described by Marin et al. The aortic body and iliac extender limbs have been designed to achieve in situ sizing of the endograft. The aortic body and ipsilateral iliac limb are contained within the same 21F delivery system that has a high level of flexibility. The contralateral iliac limb is deployed with a 19F system. The delivery systems are retracted in a controlled, incremental fashion to facilitate precise deployment. Once the aortic body of the endograft is deployed, the length of the iliac limbs can be adjusted to provide optimal exclusion of the iliac aneurysmal component while preserving flow to the internal iliac artery. Aortic necks up to 32 mm and iliac arteries up to 20 mm may be treated with the Quantum endovascular graft.

The pivotal trial of the Cordis Quantum is currently ongoing. It has received approval for marketing in the European Union. The results of the phase I FDA trial have been published.[20] Twenty-nine patients were enrolled in the trial, and graft deployment was successfully performed in all patients. There were no deaths, graft thrombosis, graft migration, aneurysm rupture, conversion to conventional aneurysm repair, or attachment site endoleaks. Seven patients experienced type 2 endoleaks. It was concluded from the trial that the Quantum graft could be safely implanted for the treatment of AAAs.

ENDOLOGIX POWERLINK SYSTEM

The Endologix PowerLink system is a one-piece bifurcated graft composed of PTFE supported by nitinol. The one-piece design eliminates the risk of endoleaks seen at attachment sites in modular devices. In addition, the frame is composed of a self-expanding non-nitinol wire, which eliminates the need for sutures to hold individual stents in place. The graft is thin-walled PTFE, which may allow for downsizing of the delivery system. The PTFE fabric is sewn to the stents only at the proximal and distal ends of the device. This allows the fabric to move off the endoskeleton. Aortic necks up to 26 mm may be treated.

In the pivotal FDA trial, 118 patients were enrolled.[21] Device deployment was performed successfully in 115 (97%). Four patients required conversion to conventional repair. Perioperative mortality was 0.8%. Endoleaks were noted in 16%, of which 10% resolved spontaneously. In addition, 2 graft limb thromboses occurred and 1 graft migration.

BAXTER LIFEPATH DEVICE

The Baxter Lifepath stent graft has evolved in design from the original White-Yu GAD endovascular device.[22] It is composed of 3 individual units, which are the main aortic body and 2 iliac limb prostheses. Each component is constructed from woven polyester and annealed Elgiloy stent wires. The graft is unique in that it is deployed by balloon expansion. Delivery of the stent graft is achieved by using 3 separate primary units. The main aortic body is deployed through a 21F sheath, and the contralateral iliac limb through a 16F sheath. Proximal aortic necks up to 27 mm and iliac implantation zones up to 15 mm may be treated. The Baxter Lifepath has been evaluated in a clinical trial in which 79 patients were enrolled. Device deployment was successful in 95%, and aortic rupture occurred in 1 patient during deployment. Immediate conversion to conventional repair was required in 2 patients. No late ruptures have been observed. The endoleak rate is 5%, with follow-up ranging from 6 months to 3 years.

ANACONDA SYSTEM

The Anaconda stent-graft system for aneurysm treatment is a fully modular system made of woven material one-third thinner than conventional graft material. The stents are made of nitinol. A unique feature is the proximal ring stent, which is composed of multiple turns of nitinol wire. The hoop strength that results from the radial force of this ring stent allows the proximal end to anchor to the aortic wall. Because of the saddle configuration of the proximal ring stent, the device can be placed so that the graft is situated at and above the renal ostia while the renal ostia themselves are uncovered. A system of magnets is used to aid in cannulating the main body of the graft to position the contralateral limb in place. Because it is a fully modular system, there is a theoretic increased risk of type 3 endoleaks because of the increase in number of articulations between pieces. This device is also currently undergoing clinical trials.

GUIDANT/EVT ANCURE DEVICE

The Guidant Ancure stent graft requires special mention. Originally designed and produced by Endovascular Technologies, the Ancure endograft system was the first stent graft to be produced commercially. Phase I and II clinical trials of the device were completed, and it received FDA approval in 1999. Initial reports found the device to be generally safe and efficacious.[23,24] However, subsequent review of the data relating to the use of the Ancure graft revealed significant difficulties associated with the delivery and deployment of the device. These difficulties resulted in considerable morbidity and in mortality in a significant number of cases. In addition, the Guidant

Corporation misrepresented the results of the stent graft use to the FDA. As a result, the device has now been withdrawn from use.

COMPARATIVE ANALYSIS

While most stent grafts are similar in the overall concept of their design, there is considerable variation of graft specifications. The endovascular devices vary in the type of stent used. Longer, stiffer stents make accommodation of angulated proximal implantation zones more challenging and may contribute to proximal attachment site endoleaks or kinking of the stent graft if it is deployed in tortuous vessels. The type and thickness of the graft material used also vary. Dacron fabric of varying porosities is the most commonly used material, although PTFE is also used. Variation in graft material may affect pressure transmission through the stent graft and may affect the tissue reaction in the perigraft material. The perigraft response may influence tissue incorporation and aneurysm sac reduction. The longitudinal stiffness of the devices also varies significantly and affects the ability of the delivery system to manage tortuosity of the iliac access vessels. Difficulty may be encountered in advancing stiffer stent grafts and delivery systems through tortuous access vessels.

Direct comparison between specific endovascular stent-graft types has been performed infrequently. One single-center experience has reported variation in the prevalence of endoleak and in change in aneurysm sac size.[25] The Zenith, Talent, Excluder, AneuRx, and Ancure devices were each evaluated. Graft limb occlusion was shown to be highest in the patients treated with the Ancure device. Type 2 endoleaks were significantly higher in the patients treated with the Excluder device, and sac shrinkage was less common with this device. Aneurysm sac enlargement occurred more commonly in patients treated with the Zenith stent graft outside the original Zenith clinical trial protocol. Patients in this group also had the highest rate of graft component separation. Aneurysm sac shrinkage was observed most commonly in patients treated with the Zenith graft as part of the multicenter trial protocol, and in patients treated with the Talent stent graft. Importantly, there was no significant difference between device types in freedom from aneurysm rupture, with an overall rate of 98.7% freedom at 24 months' follow-up. In addition, no statistically significant differences were demonstrated in secondary procedures, conversion to open repair, or migration. It is difficult to extrapolate conclusions from the results achieved in this single center, but the data are provocative and highlight the need for additional comparative analyses between stent-graft types.

SUMMARY

Endovascular treatment of AAAs has been undergoing evaluation in the clinical setting since 1991.[26] The techniques have been carried out at various centers in the United States and abroad with considerable success. When the AAA is successfully treated by endovascular means, a reduction in diameter is frequently observed. Significant reductions in major morbid events have been seen with endovascular treatment of AAAs as compared with conventional open surgery. In addition, endovascular devices provide a means of treating patients whose comorbid illnesses make conventional open repair difficult or impossible.

Selection of the specific type of stent graft for use takes into consideration a wide range of factors. Transrenal fixation such as that provided by the Zenith, Talent, and Quantum grafts may be advantageous when the proximal aortic neck is short or angulated. Controlled incremental graft deployment may also be advantageous when precise placement of the stent graft is necessary; the AneuRx, Zenith, Talent, and Quantum grafts use this method of deployment. The diameter of the delivery system and the requirement for an additional sheath to deliver the graft may be significant factors when the iliac access vessels are small or have significant occlusive disease. Lower profile delivery systems and those that possess greater flexibility can limit the potential for iliac trauma or morbidity. Migration of the stent graft can lead to the development of an endoleak at the graft attachment sites, leading to arterial perfusion of the aneurysm sac and the potential for rupture. Grafts that possess hooks or barbs to enhance fixation, including the Excluder, Zenith, and Quantum devices, may reduce the potential for migration.

Other potentially advantageous features include the ability to adjust the iliac limb length during graft deployment, as featured in the AneuRx, Zenith, and Quantum grafts. The ability to interchange device components throughout all graft sizes, such as the Zenith and Quantum grafts possess, is also useful in planning AAA repair. The ability to custom fabricate the stent graft to accommodate an individual patient's anatomic requirements, as with the Talent graft, may be advantageous when unusual anatomic characteristics are present. Similarly, the option of an aortouni-iliac configuration that is available in the Talent and Zenith grafts may be useful in patients with one occluded iliac artery. The eventual patient criteria for the use of a specific endovascular device in the treatment of AAAs will need to be more completely defined as additional clinical experience is gained and the long-term results of prospective, randomized trials are evaluated.

REFERENCES

1. Reilly JM, Tilson MD: Incidence and etiology of abdominal aortic aneurysms. *Surg Clin North Am* 69:705-711, 1989.
2. Melton L, Bickerstaff L, Hollier L, et al: Changing incidence of abdominal aortic aneurysms: A population-based study. *Am J Epidemiol* 120:379-386, 1984.
3. Lillienfeld D, Grunderson P, Sprafka J, et al: The epidemiology of abdominal aortic aneurysms: Mortality trends in the United States 1951-1980. *Atherosclerosis* 7:637-643, 1987.
4. Moore WS: Endovascular grafting technique, in Yao JST, Pearce WH (eds): *Aneurysms: New Findings and Treatments*. Norwalk, Conn, Appleton and Lange, 1995, pp 333-340.
5. Dubost C, Allary M, Oeconomos N: Resection of aneurysm of abdominal aorta: Reestablishment of continuity by preserved human arterial graft, with result after five months. *Arch Surg* 64:405-408, 1952.
6. Ernst CB: Abdominal aortic aneurysm. *N Engl J Med* 328:1167-1172, 1993.
7. National Center for Health Statistics: *Vital Statistics of the United States, 1988. Vol 2: Mortality. Part A*. Washington, DC, Government Printing Office, DHHS Publication No (PHS) 91-11010, 1991.
8. Ingoldby CJ, Wujanto R, Mitchell JE: Impact of vascular surgery on community mortality from ruptured aortic aneurysms. *Br J Surg* 73:551-553, 1986.
9. Johansson G, Swedenborg J: Ruptured abdominal aortic aneurysms: A study of incidence and mortality. *Br J Surg* 73:101-103, 1986.
10. Thomas PR, Stewart RD: Abdominal aortic aneurysm. *Br J Surg* 75:733-736, 1988.
11. Breckwoldt WL, Mackey WC, O'Donnell TF Jr: The economic implications of high-risk abdominal aortic aneurysms. *J Vasc Surg* 13:798-804, 1991.
12. Pasch AR, Ricotta JJ, May AG, et al: Abdominal aortic aneurysm: The case for elective resection. *Circulation* 70:I14S, 1984.
13. Moore WS: Transfemoral endovascular repair of abdominal aortic aneurysm: Feasibility study of the EGS system, in Parodi JC, Veith FJ, Marin ML (eds): *Endovascular Grafting Techniques*. St Louis, Quality Medical Publishing, 1995, pp 234-256.
14. Kritpracha B, Pigott JP, Russell TE, et al: Bell-bottom aortoiliac endografts: An alternative that preserves pelvic blood flow. *J Vasc Surg* 35:874-881, 2002.
15. Zarins CK, White RA, Schwarten D, et al: AneuRx stent graft versus open surgical repair of abdominal aortic aneurysms: Multicenter prospective clinical trial. *J Vasc Surg* 29:292-308, 1999.

16. Zarins CK: The US AneuRx Clinical Trial: 6-Year clinical update 2002. *J Vasc Surg* 37:904-908, 2003.

17. Matsumura JS, Brewster DC, Makaroun MS, et al: A multicenter controlled clinical trail of open versus endovascular treatment of abdominal aortic aneurysm. *J Vasc Surg* 37:262-271, 2003.

18. Greenberg RK, Lawrence-Brown M, Bhandari G, et al: An update on the Zenith endovascular graft for abdominal aortic aneurysms: Initial implantation and mid-term follow-up data. *J Vasc Surg* 33:S157-S164, 2001.

19. Faries PL, Brener BJ, Connelly TL, et al: A multicenter experience with the Talent endovascular graft for the treatment of abdominal aortic aneurysms. *J Vasc Surg* 35:1123-1128, 2002.

20. Brener BJ, Faries PL, Connelly T, et al: An *in situ* adjustable endovascular graft for the treatment of abdominal aortic aneurysms. *J Vasc Surg* 35:114-119, 2002.

21. Carpenter JP: Multicenter trial of the PowerLink bifurcated system for endovascular aortic aneirysm repair. *J Vasc Surg* 36:1129-1137, 2002.

22. White GH, Yu W, May J, et al: Three-year experience with the White-Yu endovascular GAD graft for transluminal repair of aortic and iliac aneurysms. *J Endovasc Surg* 4:124-136, 1997.

23. Moore WS, Matsumura JS, Makaroun MS, et al: Five-year interim comparison of the Guidant bifurcated endograft with open repair of abdominal aortic aneurysm. *J Vasc Surg* 38:46-55, 2003.

24. Jacobowitz GR, Lee AM, Riles TS: Immediate and late explantation of endovascular aortic grafts: The Endovascular Technologies experience. *J Vasc Surg* 29:309-316, 1999.

25. Ouriel K, Clair D, Greenberg RK, et al: Endovascular repair of abdominal aortic aneurysms: Device-specific outcome. *J Vasc Surg* 37:991-998, 2003.

26. Parodi JC, Palmaz JC, Barone HD: Transfemoral intraluminal graft implantation for abdominal aortic aneurysms. *Ann Vasc Surg* 5:491-499, 1991.

CHAPTER 6

Branched and Fenestrated Stent-Grafts for Endovascular Aortic Reconstruction

Nicholas J. Morrissey, MD
Assistant Professor of Surgery, Columbia/Weill Cornell Division of Vascular Surgery, New York, NY

Endovascular aortic techniques and devices have evolved significantly since Parodi[1] first described endovascular abdominal aortic aneurysm (AAA) repair in 1991. Anatomic challenges have made it impossible to treat all aortic aneurysms with currently available device designs. Perhaps most challenging is the inability to obtain adequate fixation between the graft and the arterial wall in cases of short and angulated aortic necks. The development of devices with fenestrations or branches to allow coverage of larger segments of the aorta while maintaining perfusion to critical branch vessels seems an attractive solution to the problems posed by short, difficult aortic necks. Devices with fenestrations and branches may be more challenging to deploy, requiring extensive experience with aortic as well as visceral and renal artery endovascular interventions. Fenestrated and branched endografts can be used in the pararenal and paravisceral aorta, the aortic arch, and at the iliac artery bifurcation to allow coverage of diseased segments of the arteries while maintaining perfusion of these critical branches.

ABDOMINAL AORTA

Since infrarenal AAA represents the largest percentage of lesions presenting for treatment, it is not surprising that branch vessel technology has focused heavily on dealing with challenging pararenal

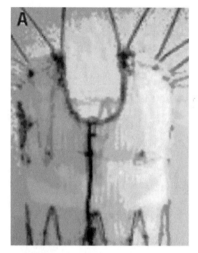

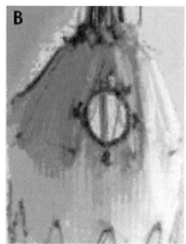

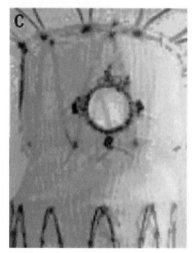

FIGURE 1.

A, Scalloped edge of stent-graft to allow continued perfusion of critical branch vessel. **B** and **C,** Fenestration in stent-graft with constrained suprarenal bare stent **(B)** and deployed bare stent **(C).** The fenestration is interrogated and a bare stent deployed in the branch vessel after deployment of the entire device.

neck anatomy.[2,3] Design of devices varies from scalloped edges at the proximal aspect of a covered stent-graft (Fig 1, *A*) to preconstructed fenestrations (Fig 1, *B* and *C*). The devices developed by Cook, Inc, are the most widely used in Australia and Europe.[2,4] Currently fenestrated stent grafts are being placed under investigational device exemptions with Food and Drug Administration–sponsored clinical trials not yet underway.

Fenestrated stent-grafts are custom fabricated for each case. In the case of the scalloped edge stent-graft, the device is positioned to place the scallop at the orifice of the critical branch, allowing perfusion of this artery, while the remaining aorta in the vicinity is covered by the device. The scallop is oriented to the vessel origin by the presence of radiopaque markers at its periphery, allowing radiographic alignment of the fenestration to the arterial origin. Devices with complete fenestrations are constructed specifically for each case. The main graft is only partially deployed so that it can be freely positioned to allow precise alignment of the fenestration with the critical branch vessel. The fenestrations have radiopaque markers at the 12-, 3-, 6-, and 9-o'clock positions to ensure precise positioning.[5] After proper positioning, the fenestrations are interrogated with wires that are advanced into the branch vessel. Balloons are placed into the branch ostia and inflated before device deployment, to maintain the position of the fenestrations as the main body conforms to the aorta.[5] Bare stents are then placed over the wires into the branch vessels and deployed (Figs 2 and 3). Anderson and col-

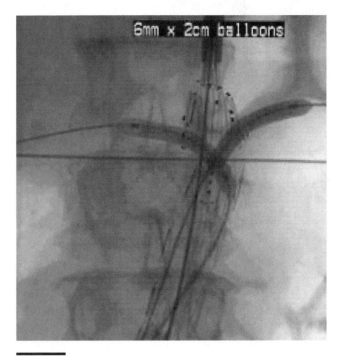

FIGURE 2.

Angioplasty balloons in the renal arteries maintain position of the fenestrations while the remainder of the graft is deployed. (Courtesy of Anderson JL, Berce M, Hartley DE: Endoluminal aortic grafting with renal and superior mesenteric artery incorporation by graft fenestration. *J Endovasc Ther* 8:3-15, 2001. Reprinted with permission.)

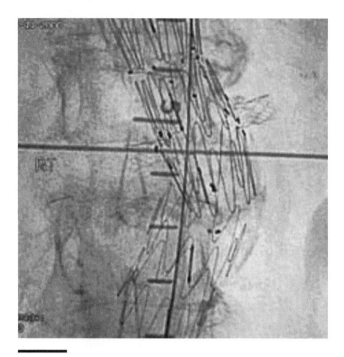

FIGURE 3.

Aortic device fully deployed and bare stents in renal arteries to maintain renal perfusion. (Courtesy of Anderson JL, Berce M, Hartley DE: Endoluminal aortic grafting with renal and superior mesenteric artery incorporation by graft fenestration. *J Endovasc Ther* 8:3-15, 2001. Reprinted with permission.)

leagues[4,5] have used this device to treat 50 patients. There was one type 1 endoleak at a fenestration at 1-year follow-up that was successfully treated with endovascular techniques. Greenberg and colleagues[3] successfully treated 22 patients with short or challenging infrarenal aortic necks with fenestrated endografts. There were no aneurysm-related deaths, and the endoleak rate was 4.5%. Three patients developed transient renal insufficiency, and 4 secondary interventions were required.[3] An example of a complex aortic aneurysm treated with a combination of a Cook fenestrated endograft and a Jomed covered stent is shown in Figure 4. Other branch vessel devices are under development. Dr Michael Marin has developed a branched pararenal graft to allow implantation of a covered stent with renal branches into the pararenal aorta. This device, being further developed by Cordis Endovascular, has the advantage of being one piece and avoiding the potential for disruption at overlap points between the main device and the branch grafts.

The experience with fenestrated endografts for infrarenal AAA is limited at this time. Early results are encouraging with respect to initial success and prevention of endoleaks in challenging aortic neck anatomy. Improvement in devices and refinement of techniques will be needed to ensure widespread applicability and success. Properly designed clinical trials involving multiple centers nationally are needed to ensure the safety and widespread applicability of these complex devices. Deployment and design of appropriate fenestrated stent-grafts requires significantly greater skill than simple infrarenal aortic grafting. Expertise in complex aortic endovascular techniques as well as percutaneous renal and visceral artery intervention is required.

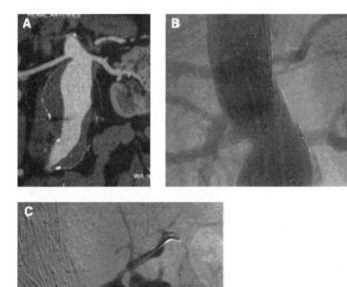

FIGURE 4.

Complex AAA with short angulated neck. Treatment involved an endograft with 4 fenestrations for the renal, superior mesenteric, and celiac arteries. An endoleak from the left renal artery was treated with a covered Jomed stent. (Courtesy of Anderson JL, Berce M, Hartley DE: Endoluminal aortic grafting with renal and superior mesenteric artery incorporation by graft fenestration. *J Endovasc Ther* 8:3-15, 2001. Reprinted with permission.)

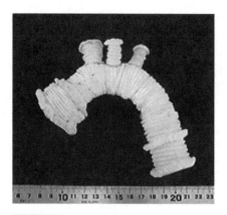

FIGURE 5.
Branched aortic arch stent-graft designed by Inoue.

ILIAC ARTERY BRANCH GRAFTS

Iliac artery involvement in patients with AAA is relatively common. In cases of bilateral iliac artery aneurysms, it may be necessary to occlude one or both of the internal iliac arteries to successfully exclude the aneurysm. While interruption of one or both internal iliac arteries may be well tolerated, the rate of buttock claudication is significant.[6] Sexual dysfunction and other forms of pelvic ischemia may also result from bilateral hypogastric artery interruption. Internal iliac artery revascularization techniques and bell-bottom stent-grafts are 2 possible methods to deal with complex iliac artery aneurysms. Stent-grafts with branches to perfuse the internal and external iliac arteries simultaneously have been developed to address iliac artery aneurysms. As in the case of aortic fenestrated stent-grafts, devices designed by Cook, Inc, and by Dr Michael Marin of Mount Sinai Medical Center in New York are examples of current technology. Such devices have been used successfully to treat complex iliac artery lesions, preserving hypogastric artery flow while successfully excluding common iliac artery aneurysms.

AORTIC ARCH BRANCH DEVICES

Aneurysms involving the aortic arch and descending aorta frequently require a 2-stage procedure involving sternotomy followed by thoracotomy. Endovascular treatment of descending thoracic aneurysms with acceptable anatomy has been described in numerous series. Application of fully endovascular techniques to aortic arch lesions requires development of branch vessel devices. A device designed by Inoue[7] has been used to treat lesions of the aortic arch with encouraging results. The device (Fig 5) can be placed in the arch and the individual branches introduced into each of the great vessels. Each device is custom designed for a particular case. More recently, Chuter and Dake[8] have developed a branch graft device for treating aortic arch lesions. They have noticed significant motion of the device with cardiac pulsations, and also caution about the risk of stroke with manipulations in the aortic arch.[8] In spite of early concerns, there is good reason to be optimistic about endovascular treatment of aortic arch pathology with branched stent-grafts.

SUMMARY

Since the advent of endovascular aortic therapy, it has been clear that treatment of more complex lesions would require more advanced technology. We are now seeing the development of devices designed to treat challenging aortic and iliac artery anatomy. The techniques required to deploy and design these devices are complicated and involve numerous areas of expertise. As devices evolve, so must the skill level of those who wish to perform these procedures. Extensive experience with aortic endografting as well as renal, visceral, and arch vessel interventions will be mandatory to ensure successful treatment of these lesions. Fenestrated and branched stent-grafts represent the next generation of devices and should allow the endovascular treatment of a greater number of patients with complex aneurysmal disease.

REFERENCES

1. Parodi JC, Palmaz JC, Barone HD: Transfemoral intraluminal graft implantation for abdominal aortic aneurysms. *Ann Vasc Surg* 5:491-499, 1991.
2. Stanley BM, Semmens JB, Lawrence-Brown MM, et al: Fenestration in endovascular grafts for aortic aneurysm repair: New horizons for preserving blood flow in branch vessels. *J Endovasc Ther* 8:16-24, 2001.
3. Greenberg R, Haulon S, Lyden S, et al: The endovascular management of juxtarenal aneurysms with fenestrated endovascular grafting. *J Vasc Surg* 39:279-287, 2004.
4. Anderson JL, Berce M, Hartley DE: Endoluminal aortic grafting with renal and superior mesenteric artery incorporation by graft fenestration. *J Endovasc Ther* 8:3-15, 2001.
5. Anderson JL: Fenestrated and branch aortic stent-grafts. *Endovascular Today* :3S-6S, 2004.
6. Mehta M, Veith F, Ohki T, et al: Unilateral and bilateral hypogastric interruption during aortoiliac aneurysm repair in 154 patients: A relatively innocuous procedure. *J Vasc Surg* 33:27-32, 2001.

7. Inoue K, Hosokawa H, Iwase T, et al: Aortic arch reconstruction by transluminally placed endovascular branched stent graft. *Circulation* 100:II-316S-321S, 1999.

8. Chuter TAM, Dake M: Ascending thoracic aortic endovascular grafting. *Endovascular Today* :10S-12S, 2004.

CHAPTER 7

Treatment of Acute and Chronic Venous Thrombotic and Occlusive Disease

Rajeev Dayal, MD
Fellow in Vascular Surgery, Department of Surgery, Division of Vascular Surgery, The New York-Presbyterian Hospital, Weill Medical College of Cornell University, New York, NY

Michael B. Silva, Jr, MD, FACS
Professor of Surgery and Radiology, Department of Surgery, Division of Vascular Surgery and Vascular Interventional Radiology, Texas Tech University Health Sciences Center, Lubbock, Texas

Symptomatic deep venous thrombosis (DVT) is a common disorder affecting 250,000 persons in the United States per year.[1] Many risk factors exist for the development of DVT; these risk factors fall into the groupings of Virchow's triad of endothelial injury, stasis, and hypercoagulable states. Risk factors include immobilization or postoperative states, spinal injury, trauma, malignancy, pregnancy or the postpartum state, the use of oral contraceptives, hypercoagulable states, and a previous episode of DVT. The standard treatment of venous thrombosis is anticoagulation, which is 98% effective in preventing recurrent DVT and pulmonary embolism. However, standard anticoagulant therapy may not prevent the development of the postthrombotic syndrome (PTS). In addition and occasionally, the symptomatology associated with critical venous occlusive and thrombotic disorders is severe, and patients may develop life- and limb-threatening complications such as phlegmasia cerulea dolens or superior vena cava syndrome. While invasive endovascular treatments for conventional DVT are controversial, the standard medical therapy for critical venous occlusive and thrombotic disorders is frequently inadequate.

Lower extremity DVT usually begins in the calf veins and may subsequently propagate to more proximal veins. It can be silent or symptomatic. Factors that impact the development of symptoms include the extent of thrombosis, the presence of collateral veins, and the degree of venous occlusion caused by the DVT. Anticoagulation remains the mainstay of treatment and prevents thrombus propagation, allows for endogenous lysis, and reduces the chance of recurrent thrombosis. However, approximately 50% of patients treated with anticoagulation continue to have abnormal findings on venous ultrasound examination 1 year after treatment initiation.[2]

Damage to the valves in the deep venous system occurs with DVT, which in turn leads to valvular incompetence. This results in venous reflux and hypertension, the consequence of which can be PTS, characterized by pain, heaviness, and edema exacerbated by walking or standing. Clinical findings include chronic skin ulceration, stasis dermatitis, hyperpigmentation, lipodermatosclerosis, and eczema. There does not, however, appear to be a strong correlation between the degree of thrombosis and the severity of the PTS.[3] Valvular incompetence is not the sole contributor to the development of PTS. Additional etiologic factors include residual venous stenoses or occlusions, as well as incompetent collateral and perforating veins. Failure of a thrombosed venous segment to recanalize is an example of the former. In a study by Prandoni et al,[4] the incidence of severe PTS was 9% at 5 years in patients with symptomatic DVT; however, patients with recurrent DVT had a 6-fold increase in the rate of PTS.[4] The mainstay of treatment for PTS is supportive and consists of graduated compression stockings, leg elevation, and behavioral modification.

A separate but uncommon late consequence of extensive ileofemoral thrombosis is the syndrome of venous claudication, characterized by leg pain and exacerbated by exercise. The etiology of venous claudication is venous hypertension secondary to residual ileofemoral venous obstruction.[5] Baseline venous hypertension is further exacerbated by the increase in blood flow that accompanies walking.

TREATMENT OF ACUTE DVT

Anticoagulation with intravenous unfractionated heparin for 3 to 5 days followed by oral warfarin for 6 months has been the traditional method of treating patients with diagnosed DVT. Newer regimens that use low molecular weight heparin have demonstrated equivalent efficacy compared to treatment with unfractionated heparin.[6] However, despite prompt and adequate anticoagulation, a significant percentage of patients treated in this conventional manner will still eventually develop venous valvular insufficiency and PTS. Valvular insufficiency has been reported to affect 28% of DVT patients at 5 years.[4] This fact has led to the hypothesis that more aggressive dissolution of thrombus might lessen the incidence of PTS. This can be accomplished with several treatment modalities, including surgical and percutaneous mechanical thrombectomy or systemic or catheter-directed thrombolysis. The rationale for a more aggressive approach is that rapid thrombus removal will resolve acute symptoms and also prevent the destruction of venous valves and the formation of late obstructive lesions that lead to the development of PTS.

The indications for intervention vary depending on the aggressiveness of the interventionalist. These indications include extensive thrombus burden or symptoms in a young patient, thrombus in the inferior vena cava (IVC), floating thrombus, phlegmasia cerulea dolens, propagation of DVT despite adequate anticoagulation, and underlying structural abnormalities such as those associated with May-Thurner syndrome. Interventions are considered more frequently in young, functional patients with acute DVT. However, invasive treatment of DVT is indicated even in the setting of severe comorbid illness for conditions such as the impending venous gangrene associated with phlegmasia cerulea dolens. This clinical scenario is characterized by arterial ischemia secondary to venous outflow obstruction, which progresses to limb loss without urgent surgical or percutaneous thrombectomy or thrombolysis.

Surgical thrombectomy was the mainstay of interventional management of DVT before the introduction of endovascular techniques. Because of the morbidity of operative interventions and the high probability of recurrence, the indication for surgical thrombectomy was limited to extensive ileofemoral DVT with limb-threatening ischemia caused by venous obstruction. Surgical thrombectomy can be coupled with a distal arteriovenous fistula to aid in maintaining patency of the treated vein. Surgical thrombectomy is an effective treatment of the acute symptoms associated with phlegmasia cerulea dolens; however, variable patency rates ranging from 42% to 84% have been reported, with rates of valvular incompetence ranging from 20% at 5 years to 44% at 10 years.[7-9]

Both systemic and catheter-directed thrombolysis have been used to treat acute DVT. The clinical success of systemic thrombolysis has been reported to be as high as 66%[10]; however, the risk of hemorrhage is significant. With systemic thrombolysis, rates of intracranial hemorrhage range from 1% to 3%, and consequently this technique has not gained widespread acceptance.[11]

As a result, catheter-directed thrombolysis has become the preferred method when invasive therapy is chosen for the treatment of acute DVT. This technique can be used to infuse high doses of thrombolytic agent directly into the vessel containing the thrombus, while minimizing systemic exposure. The largest available report of this technique is from the National Venous Thrombolysis Registry.[12] This database contains the results of treatment of 303 limbs in 287 patients, all with symptomatic lower extremity DVT. Patients treated included 221 with ileofemoral and 79 with femoral-popliteal DVT, and urokinase was used in all. Complete lysis was achieved in 31% of limbs, 50% to 99% lysis was achieved in 52% of limbs, and less than 50% lysis was achieved in 17% of limbs. Major bleeding complications were noted in 11% of patients, and pulmonary emboli developed in 1% of patients. After 1 year, the primary patency for all patients was 60%. The patency rates for patients who had complete, 50% to 99%, and less than 50% lysis were 79%, 58%, and 32%, respectively. In patients in whom complete lysis was achieved, the rate of valvular reflux was 28%. The findings demonstrated that thrombolytic therapy is more effective in thromboses that are acute or less than 4 weeks old.[13] It remains unclear whether to use IVC filters in patients with extensive DVT who are undergoing thrombolysis. Pulmonary emboli can occur with catheter-directed manipulation, but these emboli are usually small and are not of clinical significance. In the situation of a free-floating thrombus in the IVC or in patients with comorbid cardiovascular illness, the use of permanent or temporary IVC filtration devices seems warranted.[14,15]

ACCESS SITE

The access site is determined by location of the DVT, with popliteal or lesser saphenous access required for femoral thrombus, femoral access for iliac and caval thrombus, and brachial access for subclavian and innominate thrombus. The use of ultrasound in conjunction with micropuncture cannulation techniques diminishes the chance of injuring surrounding structures and causing bleeding before thrombolysis is initiated. Ideally, ipsilateral access upstream from the thrombus is preferred, although contralateral femoral access may also be used (although the presence of venous valves makes it difficult, if not impossible to cannulate vessels in a retrograde fashion). Ipsilateral popliteal vein access allows for easier traversal of popliteal, femoral, and iliac venous lesions and also allows treatment of thrombi in the IVC as well. Initially, a 5F sheath is placed and a diagnostic venogram is obtained. Occluded segments are typically crossed by using "stiff" 0.035-in hydrophilic angled glidewires (Terumo, Somerset, NJ) in combination with a 5F angled glide catheter (Angiodynamics, Queensbury, NY). A complete set of preintervention images is required to fully evaluate the extent of occluded segments, visualize collateral veins, and image the vessels downstream from the thrombus (Fig 1).

THROMBOLYTIC TECHNIQUE

A multi–side-hole infusion catheter is placed across the thrombus, as end-hole catheters do not permit efficient thrombolysis to occur. Several different infusion catheters exist including the Mewissen (Boston Scientific, Natick, Mass), Cragg-McNamara (Micro Therapeutics, Irvine, Calif), and the Proinfusion system (Angiodynamics). A catheter is chosen that is sufficiently long that it traverses the segment to be treated. Multiple thrombolytic agents can be used, with the 2 more common being urokinase (UK, Abbokinase, Abbott Labs, Chicago, Ill) and tissue plasminogen activator (TPA, alteplase, Genentech, San Francisco, Calif). The dosing regimen for urokinase consists of 240,000 units per hour for the first 4 hours, followed by an infusion of 120,000 units per hour thereafter. TPA is administered as a 1- to 2-mg initial dose delivered via pulse spray, followed by 0.5 to 1 mg per hour thereafter. Intravenous heparin is administered concomitantly either via the access sheath or via peripheral access to maintain the partial thromboplastin time at 1.5 to 2.0 times control when using urokinase, and less than 1.5 times control when using TPA.[16] Patients are typically observed in monitored settings, but usually do not require observation in an intensive care unit. Repeat venography is usually undertaken 4 to 12 hours after the institution of treatment, and if thrombolysis results in complete resolution, the procedure is terminated. If thrombolysis is incomplete or an underlying lesion is identified, then adjunctive therapies consisting of additional thrombolysis, mechanical thrombectomy, or transluminal angioplasty or stent may be considered. In cases where continued thrombolysis is chosen, patients should return for follow-up venography after another 12 to 24 hours (Fig 2).

MECHANICAL THROMBECTOMY

A myriad of devices are available for mechanical thrombectomy. These can be divided into devices that rely on rotational recirculation or those that use hydrodynamic recirculation. In devices that rely on rotational recirculation, there is an impeller or basket rotat-

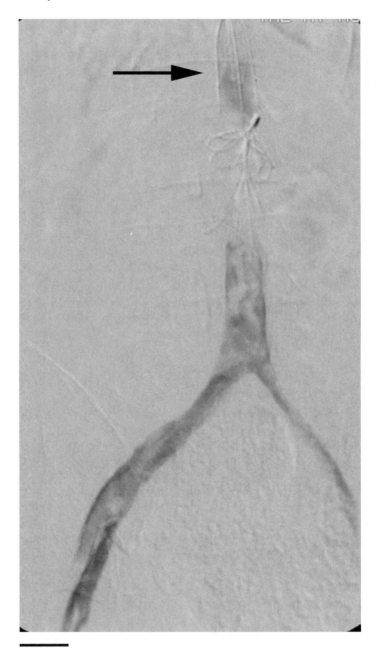

FIGURE 1.

Initial venogram obtained from popliteal approach demonstrating thrombus within iliac vein and IVC. Arrow indicates temporary filter placed above thrombus containing filter in IVC.

ing at high speed that fragments the thrombus. The resultant small particles typically embolize to the pulmonary circulation, but are too small to be of clinical significance. Examples include the Amplatz thrombectomy device (ev3, Plymouth, Minn), the PMT device (Baxter, Irvine, Calif), the Arrow-Trerotola (Arrow, Reading, Pa), the Bacchus Trellis device (Bacchus Vascular, Santa Clara, Calif), and the Cragg-Castenada thrombolytic brush (Micro Therapeutics, Irvine, Calif). The rheolytic thrombectomy devices rely on the Venturi effect to create a hydrodynamic vortex, which pulls in thrombus and causes it to fragment. The thrombectomy catheter has a separate exhaust port, which allows for evacuation of fragmented thrombus. Devices that use this form of hydrodynamic recirculation to achieve mechanical thrombectomy include the Angiojet (Possis, Minneapolis, Minn), the Oasis thrombectomy system (Boston Scientific, Natick, Mass), and the Hydrolyzer (Cordis, Warren, NJ). The primary benefit of using mechanical thrombectomy is that (1) flow may be established much more rapidly than with thrombolysis alone, and (2) the overall length of the eventual thrombolytic intervention may be shortened. These devices are most effective when used as an adjunctive method to debulk thrombus, followed by cath-

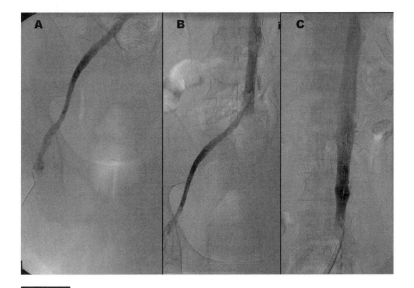

FIGURE 2.

Venogram obtained after 72 hours of thrombolysis with urokinase demonstrating recanalized **(A)** comon femoral vein, **(B)** iliac vein, and **(C)** Inferior vena cava.

eter-directed thrombolysis. Frequently, these devices will not remove thrombus that is either adherent to the vessel wall or present in a cul-de-sac or blind segment. Care must also be taken not to damage valve leaflets, and therefore, devices should be reserved for use in larger vessels, and thrombectomy should be performed as the device is advanced in the direction of blood flow. Infusion of thrombolytics has been coupled with mechanical thrombectomy. For example, 10 mg of TPA in 50 mL of normal saline can be infused through the Angiojet device and allowed to dwell for 20 minutes.[17] The thrombectomy device is then reconfigured for standard use, and mechanical thrombectomy is performed. Whether or not the addition of thrombolytics to mechanical thrombectomy produces any advantages remains to be determined.

TREATMENT OF CHRONIC DVT AND OCCLUSIVE LESIONS

The standard of care for chronic DVT and symptoms of PTS is graduated compression stockings, leg elevation, and lifestyle modification. In a select group of healthy, young patients in whom this form of treatment has failed, an endovascular option might be considered. As previously mentioned, although the pathophysiology of PTS is thought to be primarily caused by valvular incompetence, in some patients symptoms may result from obstructive thrombus.[18] Lesions within the vena cava and iliac veins may be responsive to endovascular interventions, including transluminal angioplasty and stenting.[19] Possible etiologies of chronic vena caval or iliac venous obstruction include DVT that has failed to recanalize, malignant obstruction, or the May-Thurner syndrome. Regardless of the cause, the endovascular approach consists of mechanical thrombectomy and thrombolysis, followed by angioplasty, stent, or both. Surgical reconstructions of the vena cava and iliac veins have largely been replaced by endovascular techniques.[20]

ANGIOPLASTY AND STENT

Frequently, endovascular treatment of both acute and chronic venous obstruction will reveal lesions within the vessel that are not amenable to further thrombolysis or thrombectomy. Under these circumstances, angioplasty or stenting, or both, may be useful adjuncts. Various types of stents can be used within the venous system, but self-expanding nitinol stents are preferred for the following reasons. The vessel wall is compliant, and the use of an oversized self-expanding stent lessens the risk of migration, provides more secure fixation, and diminishes the chance of perforation. Self-expanding nitinol stents also conform to the irregular contour of diseased segments more readily than do more rigid devices. Whereas the patency rates of iliac veins treated with angioplasty and stent are acceptable, the patency rates reported for angioplasty and stenting of the infrainguinal veins are less optimal and more variable. The use of stents in the treatment of infrainguinal venous disease requires further evaluation.[21]

IVC FILTERS

Fatal and nonfatal pulmonary emboli have developed as a consequence of thrombolysis,[12,14,22,23] and therefore, IVC filters may be considered in some circumstances, such as in patients with extensive thrombus of the IVC. Several retrievable caval filters are now available and can be used for this purpose. These include Recovery (CR Bard, Murray Hill, NJ), OptEase (Cordis), and the Gunther-Tulip (Cook, Bloomington, Ind). The Recovery filter received Food and Drug Administration approval for use as a removable device in August 2003; however, this filter must be placed transfemorally and, therefore, cannot be used for caval thrombosis. The Gunther-Tulip filter can be inserted either via a jugular approach or transfemorally, although it must be removed via the jugular. This filter has a hook on the cephalad portion of the device that allows its retrieval with a snare device. It is recommended that this filter be removed within 14 days of placement. Filters can be left in position for longer periods if they are adjusted to a different position to prevent the tines of the filter from becoming adherent and imbedded into the wall of the IVC.

CONCLUSION

Acute and chronic venous thrombotic and occlusive disease is responsive to percutaneous treatments including thrombolysis, thrombomechanical recanalization, venoplasty, and placement of stents. The goal of treatment for patients with acute life- or limb-threatening conditions should be the immediate relief of pain and massive edema, and resolution of ischemia. The impact of percutaneous treatments on the subsequent development of chronic venous complications, including PTS, remains to be defined. However, advances in devices and techniques have led to an increasing rate of success in the immediate dissolution of clot. Longer-term trials will eventually define which patients are appropriate candidates for interventional therapy.

REFERENCES

1. Sharafuddin MJ, Sun S, Hoballah JJ, et al: Endovascular management of venous thrombotic and occlusive diseases of the lower extremitites. *J Vasc Interv Radiol* 14:405-423, 2003.

2. Piovella F, Crippa L, Barone M, et al: Normalization rates of compression ultrasonography in patients with a first episode of deep vein thrombosis of the lower limbs: Association with recurrence and new thrombosis. *Haematologica* 87:515-522, 2002.

3. Heldal M, Seem E, Sandset PM, et al: Deep vein thrombosis: A 7-year follow-up study. *J Intern Med* 234:71-75, 1993.

4. Prandoni P, Lensing AW, Cogo A, et al: The long-term clinical course of acute deep venous thrombosis. *Ann Intern Med* 125:1-7, 1996.

5. Qvarfordt P, Eklof B, Ohlin P, et al: Intramuscular pressure, blood flow, and skeletal muscle metabolism in patients with venous claudication. *Surgery* 95:191-195, 1984.

6. Hirsh J: Low-molecular-weight heparin: A review of the results of recent studies of the treatment of venous thromboembolism and unstable angina. *Circulation* 98:1575-1582, 1998.

7. Hold M, Bull PG, Raynoschek H, et al: Deep venous thrombosis: Results of thrombectomy versus medical therapy. *Vasa* 21:181-187, 1992.

8. Meissner AJ, Huszcza S: Surgical strategy for management of deep venous thrombosis of the lower extremities. *World J Surg* 20:1149-1155, 1996.

9. Juhan CM, Alimi YS, Barthelemy PJ, et al: Late results of iliofemoral venous thrombectomy. *J Vasc Surg* 25:417-422, 1997.

10. Goldhaber SZ, Meyerovitz MF, Green D, et al: Randomized controlled trial of tissue plasminogen activator in proximal deep venous thrombosis. *Am J Med* 88:235-240, 1990.

11. Comerota AJ, Aldridge SC: Thrombolytic therapy for acute deep vein thrombosis. *Semin Vasc Surg* 5:76-81, 1992.

12. Mewissen MW, Seabrook GR, Meissner MH, et al: Catheter-directed thrombolysis for lower extremity deep venous thrombosis: Report of a national multicenter registry. *Radiology* 211:39-49, 1999.

13. Theiss W, Wirtzfeld A, Fink U, et al: The success rate of fibrinolytic therapy in fresh and old thrombosis of the iliac and femoral veins. *Angiology* 34:61-69, 1983.

14. Tarry WC, Makhoul RG, Tisnado J, et al: Catheter-directed thrombolysis following vena cava filtration for severe deep venous thrombosis. *Ann Vasc Surg* 8:583-590, 1994.

15. Lorch H, Welger D, Wagner V, et al: Current practice of temporary vena cava filter insertion: A multicenter registry. *J Vasc Interv Radiol* 11:83-88, 2000.

16. Grunwald MR, Hofmann LV: Comparison of urokinase, alteplase, and reteplase for catheter-directed thrombolysis of deep venous thrombosis. *J Vasc Interv Radiol* 15:347-352, 2004.

17. Allie DE: *Endovasc Today* 2(2):25-30, 2003.

18. Neglen P, Berry MA, Raju S: Endovascular surgery in the treatment of chronic primary and post-thrombotic iliac vein obstruction. *Eur J Vasc Endovasc Surg* 20:560-571, 2000.

19. Ing FF, Fagan TE, Grifka RG, et al: Reconstruction of stenotic or occluded iliofemoral veins and inferior vena cava using intravascular

stents: Re-establishing access for future cardiac catheterization and cardiac surgery. *J Am Coll Cardiol* 37:251-257, 2001.

20. Hurst DR, Forauer AR, Bloom JR, et al: Diagnosis and endovascular treatment of iliocaval compression syndrome. *J Vasc Surg* 34:106-113, 2001.

21. Raju S, Neglen P, Doolittle J, et al: Auxillary vein transfer in trabeculated postthrombotic veins. *J Vasc Surg* 29:1050-1064, 1999.

22. Schweizer J, Kirch W, Koch R, et al: Short- and long-term results after thrombolytic treatment of deep venous thrombosis. *J Am Coll Cardiol* 36:1336-1343, 2000.

23. Yamagami T, Kato T, Iida S, et al: Retrievable vena cava filter placement during treatment for deep venous thrombosis. *Br J Radiol* 76:712-718, 2003.

CHAPTER 8

Current Status of Gene Therapy for Intimal Hyperplasia*

Michael A. Golden, MD

Associate Professor of Surgery, University of Pennsylvania School of Medicine, Chief, Vascular Surgery, University of Pennsylvania Medical Center–Presbyterian, Philadelphia

Vascular surgery has made major advances in many areas of diagnosis and treatment of patients with vascular disease. However, the control of intimal hyperplasia and the implementation of gene therapy techniques for control of intimal hyperplasia have not experienced the same degree of progress. Intimal hyperplasia resulting in significant restenosis after angioplasty and after endarterectomy, and significant luminal narrowing after the creation of bypass anastomoses are problems that remain mainly unchecked.[1-3] As our population ages, this will become more problematic, since the prevalence of peripheral arterial occlusive disease is higher in the elderly compared with younger patients. This chapter reviews the current state of our understanding of intimal hyperplasia and its treatment by gene therapy.

BACKGROUND: INTIMAL HYPERPLASIA

At sites of arterial angioplasty, endarterectomy, bypass graft anastomoses, arteriovenous graft anastomoses, and in arterialized vein bypass grafts appears a process that is characterized by smooth muscle cell proliferation, migration, and extracellular matrix synthesis and deposition. This may combine with some degree of wall remodeling

*Supported in part by grants from the Veteran Affairs Merit Review and the National Institutes of Health–NHLBI RO1 HL56605.

and often results in luminal stenosis. This process has been studied in the laboratory with various animal models, and somewhat less stringently in rare human tissue specimens available for observational studies.[4-12] The process appears to have some common themes; however, the individual scenarios are not identical. Differentiation between them is outside the scope of this chapter, but some general themes are shared. The injury stimulus or a drastic change in biophysical properties prompts the initiation of a cascade of molecular events that ultimately results in intimal hyperplasia.[13,14] The intimal hyperplastic response is not uniformly similar between patients or even between different sites within the same patient; many factors control the degree of the intimal hyperplastic response.[3,15-17] This response is thought to be the product of interplay between mechanical forces,[18] biotransducers,[19-23] growth factors,[24-28] cytokines,[29] proteases,[5,30-32] blood-borne elements,[33,34] and the cells and connective tissue in the vessel wall.[5,35] These varied factors influencing the process of intimal hyperplasia combine to make it challenging to elucidate any single common mechanism that explains its development.

The arterial wall is composed of layers. The layer that forms the luminal surface is the intima. It is composed of endothelial cells, sometimes with some smooth muscle cells beneath the endothelium. Deep to the intima is the media, mainly composed of smooth muscle cells and extracellular matrix. The internal elastic lamina separates the intima from the media. The outermost layer of the arterial wall is the adventitia. The outer border of the media and the inner border of the adventitia is the external elastic lamina, which separates the 2 layers.

The initial events seem to include an injury or loss of functional integrity of the endothelium. This change in endothelial function may occur as increased permeability in response to toxic or inflammatory signals. Alternatively, it may be the result of actual loss of endothelial cells from the vessel luminal surface, leaving an area literally devoid of endothelium with exposure of the underlying internal elastic lamina or media to the flowing blood.[5] This allows the initiation of multiple interactions. The blood elements have been demonstrated to gain access to the vessel wall by entry between endothelial cells or by passage through regions that have been denuded of endothelial lining cells.[33,36] These invading cells are sources of cytokines and growth factors and incite recruitment of additional cells that continue the cascade that has been initiated. Monocytes[37] are key players in this activity and elaborate cytokines and growth factors. In addition, platelets that adhere to the luminal surface denuded of endothelium release mitogens and promigratory molecules.

The smooth muscle cells in the vessel wall respond to these signals and proliferate and migrate, in addition to elaborating more cytokines and growth factors. Deep to the arterial intima is the arterial media, which is a rich source of these smooth muscle cells. They proliferate in the media and also migrate into the intima and proliferate.[5] The smooth muscle cell number in the wall increases in response to this cascade, and these cells synthesize proteases and also extracellular matrix molecules such as elastin, collagen, and proteoglycans. The bulk mass of the wall increases with these events and can result in limitation of the caliber of the flow lumen. But the intima and media are not alone in the process of the arterial wall adaptation to injury. The adventitia, the outermost layer of the vessel wall, is also an active participant. Myofibroblast cells in the adventitia are activated and result in constriction of the adventitia and external elastic lamina, thereby contributing to narrowing of the entrapped vessel lumen.[38-40]

Investigators have targeted different aspects of the problem, to define better the mechanisms by which the pathologic vessel wall changes occur. For example, endothelial denudation by air-drying has been shown to result in intimal hyperplasia, as has balloon injury. Intraluminal increases in hydrostatic pressure also yield a vessel wall response.[5,41] There have also been studies demonstrating that the vessel responds to the manipulation of wall shear stress[12,19,23,42] and to alterations in wall tangential stress.[43,44]

In an effort to define opportunities for exerting control over the process of intimal hyperplasia, a large number of regulatory molecules and pathways have been specifically targeted. Some of these have shown beneficial effects in certain laboratory models of intimal hyperplasia, whereas others have not. Strategies used have included downregulation or inhibition of the production or biologic action of various molecules or factors thought to have positive regulatory influences with respect to the formation of intimal hyperplasia. Alternatively, other strategies have been focused on the upregulation or overexpression of molecules considered to be inhibitors of the process. Among others, processes thought important include smooth muscle cell proliferation and migration, thrombosis, inflammation, extracellular matrix synthesis, and vessel wall remodeling. Stimulatory molecules have been targeted for downregulation or inhibition, including growth factors such as platelet-derived growth factor,[25,45] basic fibroblast growth factor,[46-48] and transforming growth factor-β1.[28] Chemotactic factors have also been targeted, such as macrophage chemotactic protein-1.[34,49] Cell cycle molecules have also been targeted with the plan that prevention of vascular smooth muscle proliferation would inhibit the process of intimal hyperplasia.[50,51] The growth inhibitor β-interferon was also studied.[52] Strategies involving controlled cytotoxicity with spatially controlled gene transfer of a nonhuman enzyme that catalyzes the reaction for the conversion of a harmless precursor molecule into a toxic product have been used in conjunction with systemic delivery of the harmless precursor to achieve inhibition of intimal hyperplasia.[53,54] Intracellular signaling pathway targeting has also been pursued to inhibit cell proliferation.[55] Urokinase plasminogen activator has been used as a target for upregulation to inhibit the contribution of thrombosis.[32] The adjustment of extracellular matrix biology has also demonstrated an effect on wall remodeling.[56,57] There are a large number of cellular participants in the process, and many coordinated events occur to yield the dramatic and important changes of wall thickening and luminal stenosis that characterize the pathologic problem called "intimal hyperplasia."

This interplay of many actors and processes forms a complex and interwoven fabric that is difficult to understand. As such, it has proven quite difficult to determine specific regulatory relationships that will allow precise control of the pathology. Such control may be achieved best with a combined attack at multiple points in the cascade of events leading to intimal hyperplasia. This may be a very important approach, especially since certain therapeutic strategies that have demonstrated a clear beneficial effect in animal models of arterial pathology have failed to reproduce any beneficial effect when applied to human pathology.[1] This uncertainty translates into a huge problem. When the target for manipulation by gene therapy is not yet clearly defined, that results in a major deterrent to proceeding with human gene therapy trials.

It should also be emphasized that although there are many similarities in the intimal hyperplasia seen in different settings (angioplasty, endarterectomy, vein bypass, prosthetic bypass, and arteriovenous fistula), they do differ somewhat from one another. It is not clear that determining an effective method for controlling the process in one setting will guarantee successful transfer of that strategy as an effective treatment in another setting.

GENE THERAPY: PRINCIPLES AND PRACTICE

Gene therapy consists of a therapeutic intervention aimed at achieving a clinically desirable goal by means of modification of gene expression (Fig 1). Our genetic material contains a massive amount of information encoded in the sequence of nucleotides in our DNA. This is transcribed into messenger RNA (mRNA) and subsequently translated into protein. This cascade of information transfer and regulation is complex and is regulated quite stringently with positive and negative controls. The goal of gene therapy is manipulation of this genetic expression in the setting of disease to produce an improved outcome. Gene therapy alters the pattern of biologic molecules that orchestrate the function of cells, tissues, and organs.

Gene Therapy for Control of Intimal Hyperplasia

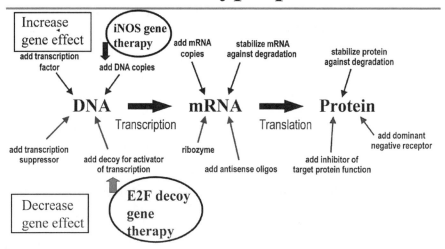

FIGURE 1.

This illustration reveals examples of methods by which the cascade of gene expression can be modified by specifically targeted gene therapy. Examples of methods to increase the expression of a selected gene are listed horizontally above the line, "DNA→mRNA→Protein," and methods to decrease gene expression are listed horizontally below this line. The *arrows* indicate the specific site of action for the individual gene therapy interventions. An example of increasing gene expression, currently included in a planned gene therapy trial to control intimal hyperplasia, is the introduction of additional copies of the inducible nitric oxide synthase *(iNOS)* gene as seen in the *uppermost circle*. Conversely, an example of decreasing gene expression, currently included in completed and ongoing gene therapy trials to control intimal hyperplasia, is the use of a transcription factor decoy for the E2F transcription factor. This is indicated in the *lower circle*.

TARGET TYPES

Possible candidate genes or molecules have been discussed above with respect to the goal of controlling the formation of intimal hyperplasia. When the decision is made to target a specific molecule, the exact plan of attack is dependent on the biology of that molecule. For example, at what point in the expression of this molecule is the gene therapy intervention most likely to be effective? The plan might be to provide added copies of the gene of interest so that it will be expressed independent of the level of native gene expression. Alternatively, intervention could be at the point of targeting the transcription factors that allow this gene to be turned on and expressed, or turned off and not expressed. There is a human gene therapy trial that is using this strategy of inhibiting the stimulating effect of a transcription factor, and the trial will be discussed in more detail below. Alternatively, after the gene has been transcribed into mRNA, the message could be targeted for interference of further processing and for destruction, such as with antisense RNA or a ribozyme that cleaves the message of interest and inactivates it. Further down the cascade of gene expression, the effect of the gene of interest could be abrogated, by introducing a dominant negative receptor construct. This dominant negative receptor would act in the place of the native receptor and bind the signaling protein but would prevent signal propagation, and thereby confer its inhibitory effect.

GENE TRANSFER SPECIFICITY

There are many ways in which the pattern of gene expression can be altered. It is important to understand the biology of the different methods, to allow the choice of strategy to embrace the specific biologic characteristics of the problem. For example, if a transcription factor approach is selected, then likely the only cells that will respond as desired are those that have been altered successfully by the gene therapy procedure. This implies that the method of gene transfer must successfully affect almost all the required cells in the tissue of interest. For example, all smooth muscle cells may need to be transduced, but not all the endothelial cells, or vice versa. Or possibly it may be helpful to target endothelial or smooth muscle cells, or both in a certain location, but not those same cell types in other sites, and also not in distant organs and unrelated tissues. For example, intravenous administration of adenovirus often results in gene transfer in the liver. This is quite helpful if the liver is the target, but if a distant artery is the target and gene transfer in the liver is not desired, then this would be a problem with intravenous delivery with adenovirus. In addition to gene transfer specificity, there is also the consideration of gene transfer efficiency.

GENE TRANSFER EFFICIENCY

The efficiency of gene transfer relates to the relative percentage of cells in the targeted tissue that actually are genetically modified with the gene transfer protocol. If all the targeted cells are transfected, then the efficiency is 100%. It is usually less uniformly successful, especially in the setting of in vivo biologic systems. In contrast, gene transfer of cells in culture is associated with much higher efficiency. Returning to our example described above of the dominant negative receptor construct gene therapy approach, this would imply the requirement for a significantly high level of gene transfer efficiency to thoroughly inhibit the effect of possible wild-type receptor stimulation. Clearly, any cell without the dominant negative receptor construct gene transfer would lack the dominant negative receptor on its surface, and would exhibit only the wild-type receptor. Such an untransduced cell, with its surface containing only the wild-type receptor, would be expected to engage in signaling unhindered when in contact with ligand. This type of strategy would require high gene transfer efficiency for success. This is in stark contrast to the situation in which a stimulatory gene with a secreted product is targeted for amplification. In the latter instance, even if much less than half the cells were successfully targeted, their secreted stimulatory product might successfully drive all the cells in the tissue to respond as desired. This would represent a much less difficult technical goal for gene transfer than requiring almost uniformly successful gene transfer throughout the target tissue. On the other hand, a secreted product of the gene transfer strategy might also induce changes that would not be confined to specific cells in the local tissue, and this concern must be taken into account in planning the treatment strategy, especially from the point of view of safety.

GENE TRANSFER DURATION

In addition to the specificity and efficiency of gene transfer, the duration of gene transfer must be considered carefully when planning a gene therapy strategy. The biology of the problem being treated and the specific gene being targeted will determine what length of gene transfer duration is desirable. Examination of the molecular mechanism of many human diseases reveals that the pathology is a result of an imbalance in the stimulatory and inhibitory regulatory mechanisms, leading to an inadequate response, an overpowering response, or a response that is prolonged in duration and fails to return to the natural baseline level of activity. With this in mind, one can appreciate that the excessive duration of a gene transfer strategy might result in the lattermost circumstance described above, whereas an inadequate response might be the product of a gene therapy strategy that had too short a duration of gene transfer effect. Clearly, for some diseases, such as for familial hypercholesterolemia, characterized by a permanent deficit in low-density lipoprotein receptor function, an effective therapeutic strategy would likely require a permanent genetic modification. The level of gene expression or effect of the transgene is a function of not only the efficiency of gene transfer and the duration of gene transfer as described above, but also the amount of expression of the transgene by the cells that are genetically modified. All of these factors are important in designing a gene therapy strategy.

TOXICITY

Another consideration that must remain in the forefront of any plan to apply gene therapy to human disease is the concern about toxicity. This may occur in many different forms. There may be direct toxicity of a viral vector itself, resulting in host cell dysfunction or death. Other forms of toxicity include possible immune response destruction of cells or tissues, or both, that had undergone successful gene transfer. In addition, inexact dosing of the gene transfer effect or varied gene expression of the target tissue might result in toxicity, as characterized by too high or too low gene expression. Additional problems might include gene transfer to cells or tissues, or both, that were not originally planned for gene transfer but that occurred secondary to the inexact ability to target only specific cells or tissues in a specific site. There might also be some nonspecific inflammation that might occur secondary to the use of viral vectors that can yield undesirable effects. Also, live viral vectors have been used in specific circumstances. This has been associated with not just concerns about safety, but in a nonvascular human trial, it has been associated with actual documented problems with toxicity and mortality.[58] With the use of live virus, potential toxicity may result from the uncontrolled replication of the live virus. Uncontrolled replication may also theoretically occur with the use of replication-deficient virus that undergoes recombination with wild-type virus and becomes replication competent. Retroviral gene transfer has been associated with incorporation of the viral DNA into the host cell DNA,[59] and this is associated with concerns about possible mutagenicity, malignancy, or other disruption in normal cell regulation. Finally, in certain applications, such as for the treatment of malignant disease,[60,61] the use of gene therapy is designed to induce cell toxicity and kill tumor cells, but in a very controlled fashion. The problem with toxicity in this type of situation may be a problem in targeting, as unintentional gene transfer to other tissues would be expected to result in undesired toxicity. With a modality as powerful as gene therapy, the issue of toxicity remains a central concern about advancing its use into human application.

SUCCESS OF REPEATED GENE TRANSFER TREATMENTS

Vascular disease is usually a multifocal disease, and also likely to be problematic repeatedly over time. This spatial and temporal pattern of disease makes quite germane the question about the ability to repeat the gene therapy treatment. For some human diseases, treatments can be used safely only once per patient. However, for the treatment of patients with vascular disease, it would be very desirable to be able to use an effective gene therapy strategy more than once and not diminish the efficacy or safety of the treatment. This is a real concern, especially with viral vectors. There is ample evidence that, much like a vaccine, exposure to the viral vector significantly inhibits the success of a subsequent attempt at achieving gene transfer with a subsequent exposure to the vector.[62]

VECTOR TYPES

Depending on the molecule of interest and the desired target, a variety of vector systems are available for use. They fall into categories of DNA or RNA that can increase or decrease the expression of the targeted gene. Then there are viral vectors that are attenuated viruses that have been genetically engineered not only to carry the gene of interest, but also to have their ability to replicate themselves be attenuated or destroyed. Finally, there are some new vector systems that use novel mechanisms, such as tat proteins to create a fusion protein with a protein of interest, which can then pass easily into cells and affect gene expression.

Naked DNA, Oligodeoxynucleotides, Plasmid DNA/DNA Liposomes and RNA Liposomes With or Without Viral Proteins

DNA does not pass through the cell membrane easily and can be degraded once internalized. It is a low-efficiency gene transfer system (<1%) and also depends on the size of the DNA molecule being delivered. The addition of pressure and hydrogel-coated balloons can improve the results.[63,64]

Complexing DNA or RNA with cationic liposomes greatly improves cellular uptake. The process, however, remains less efficient than that with viral systems. This approach with DNA or with mRNA can be used to increase the gene copy number or message number to increase the gene effect. Alternatively, DNA liposome complexes can deliver antisense oligodeoxynucleotides for inhibition of gene expression. Similarly, ribozyme (RNA) delivered to cells can cleave mRNA and result in decreased protein synthesis and effectively lower gene expression. The addition of viral proteins, such as those from the hemagglutinating virus of Japan, also increases the uptake of the nucleic acid liposome complexes via viral receptor action on the target cell membrane.[65] Like RNA, DNA is easy to engineer, does not limit transgene size, is effective for cells independent of their proliferative state, but is associated with expression that is short-term.

Retrovirus

The retrovirus was one of the first viral vectors to be used. It has a double-stranded, linear RNA genome. After the virus enters the cell, the viral genome is copied by viral-dependent DNA polymerase (reverse transcriptase) into a DNA copy, which integrates stably into the host cell DNA. This permits long-term expression since the genome is integrated into the host DNA; however, concerns about mutagenicity are associated with the integration process. The virus is relatively nonimmunogenic, and it is usually difficult to grow in high titers. The process of infection is also somewhat low efficiency and requires ongoing cell division for good yields.[66,67] Because of stable transfection, retroviral-mediated gene transfer has been used for gene transfer when ex vivo gene transfer and reimplantation of the genetically modified endothelial or smooth muscle cells are desired.[59] This strategy has been used to determine the biologic effect of overexpression of a gene of interest in the arterial wall, or to make what might be called a "designer intima."[68] Lentiviruses are a type of retrovirus and are relatively nonimmunogenic, infect cells independent of their proliferative state, and incorporate into the genome for prolonged gene expression. The human immunodeficiency virus is a lentivirus, and therefore, there are concerns about the safety of using such vectors.

Adenovirus

The adenovirus is a double-stranded DNA virus with a number of subtypes. It constitutes the agent of the "common cold" and has been well studied. It can be made replication deficient by deleting the E1 portion of the viral genome, and can be grown up in high titers. It enters cells readily without regard to their proliferative status, and does so with high efficiency via a receptor-mediated mechanism, and effectively expresses its transgene. The viral genome remains episomal and does not integrate into the host genome. This results in freedom from mutagenicity, but is also associated with transient transgene expression (1-2 weeks). The virus incites a host immune response.[62,69-71] The immunology of the adenovirus is somewhat unclear, but it appears that the viral capsid incites a host immune response even if the virus is no longer alive, making creation of an entirely nonimmunogenic adenoviral vector unlikely, although re-engineering efforts continue.

Adeno-Associated Virus

Adeno-associated virus is a DNA virus that is not associated with human disease and requires a helper virus for replication. This helper virus needs to be an adenovirus or herpesvirus, which leads to concerns about purity and contamination of the product. It is also difficult to produce in high titers, and it will accept only small transgenes. Adeno-associated virus can infect cells independent of their proliferative status, and when the virus enters the cell, the viral genome translocates to the nucleus where it incorporates into the host genome, usually at chromosome 19q. There is minimal concern about mutagenicity, and good long-term transgene expression is usually observed with this virus, which is relatively nonimmunogenic.[72-74]

Vaccinia, Herpes, or Other Viruses

There is work ongoing on other viral vectors and to harness live, attenuated viruses that are not replication deficient for use as gene therapy vectors. These viruses are DNA viruses that are showing potential for use, but more information is needed.[75,76]

New Vectors: Tat Proteins

From the human immunodeficiency virus, the tat protein moiety has been used to make fusion proteins that can rapidly and effectively pass through the cell membranes to gain access to the interior of the target cell. The mechanism of this is still under investigation, but it is remarkably effective. This allows the use of protein delivery for the modification of genetic expression and cell phenotype.[77]

ROUTES/METHODS FOR GENE TRANSFER

The selection of the method of vector delivery depends on the following features: the vector, the target tissue, and the transgene. With respect to vascular gene transfer, it is usually local gene transfer that is desired. Usually, a specific site is in need of genetic modification. It is that site, and that site alone, in which we would like to target our therapy. Presently, no vector can target specific vascular tissue when delivered systemically as an injection, intravenously, intramuscularly, or subcutaneously. Much effort has been directed toward designing the method of delivery of the vector to target the specific vascular anatomic site of interest. These methods have included intraluminal delivery of the vector, or in some cases, periadventitial delivery of the vector. Intraluminal delivery can be performed in a large artery by using a double-balloon catheter.[78] The 2 balloons are separated by an intervening catheter segment that has holes and a separate lumen. When the balloons are inflated at each end, the intervening segment of artery is isolated from the blood. The lumen of the catheter in that segment is used to empty the isolated arterial segment of blood, and then the vector solution is instilled and allowed to dwell in contact with the arterial wall. Then the solution is removed and the flow restored. In other instances, specialized balloons such as microporous balloons or channel balloons are used that allow contact between the engineered surface of the balloon and the arterial wall. Other balloon technologies allow for hydrogel-coated surfaces on balloons to be in contact with the arterial wall for a period of time before deflation and balloon removal. The balloons function by allowing the vector to pass into the arterial wall by passive diffusion, facilitated diffusion, or actual mechanical infiltration, with the latter process itself being associated with some degree of arterial wall disruption or injury.[79-82]

Periadventitial delivery of vector-containing solution has also been performed on surgically exposed arteries, with excellent results in the laboratory setting. This would clearly be an option for surgical anastomoses should it be proven clinically helpful.[83,84]

Ex vivo gene transfection of endothelial cells and smooth muscle cells is also an option. Endothelial cells, smooth muscle cells, or both can be genetically modified and then placed on the luminal surface of grafts or injured arterial segments, with reconstitution of the arterial wall with vascular cells genetically modified to exhibit specific characteristics.[68,85]

TARGETS

The sections above discussed many potential targets for intervention in the biology of the vascular wall to achieve inhibition of intimal hyperplasia. Although many potentially helpful targets can be pursued, considerations of specificity and efficacy of delivery of gene transfer vectors, combined with considerations of duration of gene transfer effect and concerns with possible toxicity and risk, have led to only a small number of human trials that might be considered to involve gene therapy. Human gene therapy trials have not been without any problems with toxicity.[58] This has prompted exquisitely strict regulation, monitoring, and restrictions on such trials in general, for the protection of human subjects. It has become more challenging and resource intensive to perform such trials. In addition, unlike some brain tumors and mesothelioma, which are diseases that have uniformly rapidly fatal outcomes, intimal hyperplasia is not uniformly guaranteed to be a problem. So the risk profile that is acceptable for human trials of gene therapy for the control of intimal hyperplasia must be limited to what might be considered less radical. In terms of human gene therapy trials that involve patients with vascular disease, there have been trials to treat patients with genetic lipid disorders[59] and patients with nonbypassable lower extremity and cardiac ischemia.[86-88] These trials do not directly impact the treatment of intimal hyperplasia and, therefore, will not be mentioned further here. The following will describe the experience to date with human gene therapy trials for the control of intimal hyperplasia.

HUMAN GENE THERAPY TRIALS FOR INTIMAL HYPERPLASIA

Two main strategies have been developed to the point of reaching the stage of human trials of gene therapy for the inhibition of intimal hyperplasia. The first strategy uses a short oligodeoxynucleotide that acts as a decoy for the E2F transcription factor involved in the regulation of smooth muscle cell proliferation in the vessel wall. The second involves the delivery of the inducible nitric oxide synthase (iNOS) gene to the vessel wall.

The first strategy (the E2F decoy strategy) has made the greatest progress as of the present. Complex regulatory systems keep the vascular smooth muscle cells in the normal vessel wall quiescent and not proliferating. During times of vessel injury, however, regulation of gene expression is drastically altered. Smooth muscle cellular proliferation in the arterial wall is regulated by a balance of positive and negative influences on proliferation. The interactions between the series of cyclin proteins, cyclin-dependent kinases, and inhibitors of cyclin-dependent kinases achieve this regulation. To shift the smooth muscle cell from quiescence to proliferation, a series of phosphorylation events occur through the cyclins and cyclin-dependent kinases, resulting in phosphorylation of retinoblastoma protein (Rb). Normally, Rb is in the unphosphorylated state, is bound to DNA elongation factor (E2F), and keeps the E2F from causing gene transcription. When arterial injury occurs, Rb becomes activated by phosphorylation and E2F is released, allowing it to interact with the DNA. At such times, the liberated E2F transcription factor binds to the gene expression regulatory site on the DNA and causes cell-cycle regulatory genes to be expressed that result in smooth muscle cell proliferation. This cascade of events, including cell proliferation, can be blocked by delivery of a decoy molecule consisting of a short chain of nucleotides that resembles the binding site on the DNA for the E2F transcription factor. The decoy binds the liberated E2F transcription factor, traps it, and prevents it from interacting with the gene DNA, thereby preventing subsequent smooth muscle cell proliferation. This strategy was shown to be effective in animal models,[89-91] and has been advanced to a series of human clinical gene therapy trials. The phase I trial was called PREVENT and was a single-center, randomized, double-blinded, prospective, controlled trial involving patients undergoing autologous vein bypass grafts for lower extremity ischemia. The vein conduit was harvested from the patient and then treated by immersing it under pressure in 1 of 3 solutions: (1) saline, (2) saline with the E2F decoy oligodeoxynucleotide, or (3) saline with a oligodeoxynucleotide consisting of a nonsense scrambled sequence of nucleotides. The bypass vein grafts were rinsed and then implanted by using standard vascular surgical techniques. The investigators were able to demonstrate approximately 80% transfection efficiency, indicating that they were able to deliver the decoy to 80% of the cells in the vein graft wall. In addition, they noted significant inhibition of smooth muscle cellular proliferation in samples of vein that received the E2F decoy compared with veins that received the other control treatments. Designed as a phase I trial to examine safety, no differences in postoperative complications were noted among the 3 groups. The trial was not powered to assess efficacy, but there appeared to be fewer graft revisions and critical stenoses noted in the E2F decoy–treated group compared with those in the control groups.[92]

The success of the phase I trial led to the phase II trial PREVENT II. In this trial, conducted in Germany, vein grafts were harvested and treated with a solution of E2F decoy versus control solution before implantation as coronary artery bypass grafts. The results of this study have been presented as an abstract and demonstrated no adverse events associated with the treatment. They demonstrated no difference in clinical end points, but there was a significant decrease in the rate of significant stenosis in the E2F-treated vein grafts compared with the control vein grafts.[93]

There has been advancement of this into a much larger phase III trial, PREVENT III. The study consists of a multicenter, randomized, blinded, prospective clinical trial examining this treatment in the setting of lower extremity, autologous vein bypass grafts for ischemia. The vein grafts were harvested and treated with the E2F-containing solution versus the control solution before implantation as vein bypass grafts. The end points of toxicity, complications, and graft stenosis, revision, failure, and patency at the end of a year will be examined. Patient recruitment has been completed in that trial, and follow-up data accrual is ongoing. The results of the study should be available relatively soon, since the postoperative follow-up for the study data accrual is only a year. The results from this trial are awaited with great excitement. This has been a pioneering endeavor in terms of recruiting a large number of participating sites to achieve adequate patient recruitment for successful completion of the study. Also, there is great optimism for this trial because the phase I and II studies had shown great promise for the treatment of vein graft stenosis, and this is a problem for which we do not currently have a good treatment by any modality.

The second gene therapy strategy that has progressed to the point of a human clinical trial for control of intimal hyperplasia involves the delivery of the iNOS gene to the vessel wall. The trial is a phase I trial to assess safety. The patient population to be studied includes patients on dialysis in need of arteriovenous prosthetic graft surgery. The vector is a replication-deficient adenovirus encoding the iNOS gene, which should result in synthesis of iNOS and release of NO to affect not only the cells that successfully received the iNOS gene transfer, but also the surrounding cells in a paracrine fashion. NO inhibits smooth muscle cell proliferation and migration, promotes endothelial cell survival and proliferation, and inhibits platelet and leukocyte adhesion. These are all highly attractive influences for stabilizing and repairing the injured vessel wall. There is strong support for this strategy from investigations in animals.[94-96] Currently, the study is still awaiting additional preclinical data, but it has attracted great interest.

It is evident from the material presented above that we have made progress, but it is still early in the attempt to control the problem of intimal hyperplasia in our patients. The pathobiology of the problem is incompletely understood, and our vectors and methods for achieving gene transfer are inexact and in need of improvement. As such, there is great opportunity for further advances to be made in this exciting and promising area.

REFERENCES

1. Karsch KR, Preisack MB, Baildon R, et al: Low molecular weight heparin (reviparin) in percutaneous transluminal coronary angioplasty. Results of a randomized, double-blind, unfractionated heparin and pla-

cebo-controlled, multicenter trial (REDUCE trial). Reduction of Restenosis After PTCA, Early Administration of Reviparin in a Double-Blind Unfractionated Heparin and Placebo-Controlled Evaluation. *J Am Coll Cardiol* 28:1437-1443, 1996.

2. Kastrati A, Schuhlen H, Hausleiter J, et al: Restenosis after coronary stent placement and randomization to a 4-week combined antiplatelet or anticoagulant therapy: Six-month angiographic follow-up of the Intracoronary Stenting and Antithrombotic Regimen (ISAR) Trial [see comments]. *Circulation* 96:462-467, 1997.

3. Bandyk DF, Kaebnick HW, Adams MB, et al: Turbulence occurring after carotid bifurcation endarterectomy: A harbinger of residual and recurrent carotid stenosis. *J Vasc Surg* 7:261-274, 1988.

4. Clowes AW, Reidy MA, Clowes MM: Mechanisms of stenosis after arterial injury. *Lab Invest* 49:208-215, 1983.

5. Clowes AW, Clowes MM, Fingerle J, et al: Regulation of smooth muscle cell growth in injured artery. *J Cardiovasc Pharmacol* 14:S12-S15, 1989.

6. Zwolak RM, Adams MC, Clowes AW: Kinetics of vein graft hyperplasia: Association with tangential stress. *J Vasc Surg* 5:126-136, 1987.

7. McCann RL, Larson RM, Mitchener JS, et al: Histological and biochemical studies of vascular autografts. *Artery* 6:267-279, 1980.

8. Westerband A, Crouse D, Richter LC, et al: Vein adaptation to arterialization in an experimental model. *J Vasc Surg* 33:561-569, 2001.

9. Westerband A, Gentile AT, Hunter GC, et al: Intimal growth and neovascularization in human stenotic vein grafts. *J Am Coll Surg* 191:264-271, 2000.

10. Woodside KJ, Naoum JJ, Torry RJ, et al: Altered expression of vascular endothelial growth factor and its receptors in normal saphenous vein and in arterialized and stenotic vein grafts. *Am J Surg* 186:561-568, 2003.

11. Lindner V, Fingerle J, Reidy MA: Mouse model of arterial injury. *Circ Res* 73:792-796, 1993.

12. Kumar A, Lindner V: Remodeling with neointima formation in the mouse carotid artery after cessation of blood flow. *Arterioscler Thromb Vasc Biol* 17:2238-2244, 1997.

13. Koyama H, Olson NE, Reidy MA: Cell signaling in injured rat arteries. *Thromb Haemost* 82:806-809, 1999.

14. Shigematsu K, Koyama H, Olson NE, et al: Phosphatidylinositol 3-kinase signaling is important for smooth muscle cell replication after arterial injury. *Arterioscler Thromb Vasc Biol* 20:2373-2378, 2000.

15. Gibson CM, Goel M, Cohen DJ, et al: Six-month angiographic and clinical follow-up of patients prospectively randomized to receive either tirofiban or placebo during angioplasty in the RESTORE trial. Randomized Efficacy Study of Tirofiban for Outcomes and Restenosis. *J Am Coll Cardiol* 32:28-34, 1998.

16. Cox JL, Chiasson DA, Gotlieb AI: Stranger in a strange land: The pathogenesis of saphenous vein graft stenosis with emphasis on structural

and functional differences between veins and arteries. *Prog Cardiovasc Dis* 34:45-68, 1991.

17. Davies MG, Hagen PO: Pathophysiology of vein graft failure: A review. *Eur J Vasc Endovasc Surg* 9:7-18, 1995.

18. Ballyk PD, Walsh C, Butany J, et al: Compliance mismatch may promote graft-artery intimal hyperplasia by altering suture-line stresses. *J Biomech* 31:229-237, 1998.

19. Meyerson SL, Skelly CL, Curi MA, et al: The effects of extremely low shear stress on cellular proliferation and neointimal thickening in the failing bypass graft. [Erratum appears in *J Vasc Surg* 34:580, 2001.] *J Vasc Surg* 34:90-97, 2001.

20. Bassiouny HS, White S, Glagov S, et al: Anastomotic intimal hyperplasia: Mechanical injury or flow induced. *J Vasc Surg* 15:708-716, 1992.

21. Kohler TR, Kirkman TR, Kraiss LW, et al: Increased blood flow inhibits neointimal hyperplasia in endothelialized vascular grafts. *Circ Res* 69: 1557-1565, 1991.

22. Kohler TR, Jawien A: Flow affects development of intimal hyperplasia after arterial injury in rats. *Arterioscler Thromb* 12:963-971, 1992.

23. Mattsson EJ, Kohler TR, Vergel SM, et al: Increased blood flow induces regression of intimal hyperplasia. *Arterioscler Thromb Vasc Biol* 17: 2245-2249, 1997.

24. Reidy MA: Neointimal proliferation: The role of basic FGF on vascular smooth muscle cell proliferation. *Thromb Haemost* 70:172-176, 1993.

25. Jawien A, Bowen-Pope DF, Lindner V, et al: Platelet-derived growth factor promotes smooth muscle migration and intimal thickening in a rat model of balloon angioplasty. *J Clin Invest* 89:507-511, 1992.

26. Golden MA, Au YP, Kirkman TR, et al: Platelet-derived growth factor activity and mRNA expression in healing vascular grafts in baboons. Association in vivo of platelet-derived growth factor mRNA and protein with cellular proliferation. *J Clin Invest* 87:406-414, 1991.

27. Mondy JS, Lindner V, Miyashiro JK, et al: Platelet-derived growth factor ligand and receptor expression in response to altered blood flow in vivo. *Circ Res* 81:320-327, 1997.

28. Wolf YG, Rasmussen LM, Ruoslahti E: Antibodies against transforming growth factor-beta 1 suppress intimal hyperplasia in a rat model. *J Clin Invest* 93:1172-1178, 1994.

29. Ascher E, Scheinman M, Hingorani A, et al: Effect of p53 gene therapy combined with CTLA4Ig selective immunosuppression on prolonged neointima formation reduction in a rat model. *Ann Vasc Surg* 14:385-392, 2000.

30. Carmeliet P, Moons L, Herbert JM, et al: Urokinase but not tissue plasminogen activator mediates arterial neointima formation in mice. *Circ Res* 81:829-839, 1997.

31. Cherr GS, Motew SJ, Travis JA, et al: Metalloproteinase inhibition and the response to angioplasty and stenting in atherosclerotic primates [see comment]. *Arterioscler Thromb Vasc Biol* 22:161-166, 2002.

32. DeYoung MB, Tom C, Dichek DA: Plasminogen activator inhibitor type 1 increases neointima formation in balloon-injured rat carotid arteries. *Circulation* 104:1972-1977, 2001.

33. Fingerle J, Johnson R, Clowes AW, et al: Role of platelets in smooth muscle cell proliferation and migration after vascular injury in rat carotid artery. *Proc Natl Acad Sci U S A* 86:8412-8416, 1989.

34. Egashira K, Zhao Q, Kataoka C, et al: Importance of monocyte chemoattractant protein-1 pathway in neointimal hyperplasia after periarterial injury in mice and monkeys. *Circ Res* 90:1167-1172, 2002.

35. Chung IM, Gold HK, Schwartz SM, et al: Enhanced extracellular matrix accumulation in restenosis of coronary arteries after stent deployment [see comment]. *J Am Coll Cardiol* 40:2072-2081, 2002.

36. Faggiotto A, Ross R, Harker L: Studies of hypercholesterolemia in the nonhuman primate: I. Changes that lead to fatty streak formation. *Arteriosclerosis* 4:323-340, 1984.

37. Westerband A, Mills JL, Marek JM, et al: Immunocytochemical determination of cell type and proliferation rate in human vein graft stenoses. *J Vasc Surg* 25:64-73, 1997.

38. Mondy JS, Williams JK, Adams MR, et al: Structural determinants of lumen narrowing after angioplasty in atherosclerotic nonhuman primates. *J Vasc Surg* 26:875-883, 1997.

39. Geary RL, Nikkari ST, Wagner WD, et al: Wound healing: A paradigm for lumen narrowing after arterial reconstruction. *J Vasc Surg* 27:96-106, 1998.

40. Geary RL, Williams JK, Golden D, et al: Time course of cellular proliferation, intimal hyperplasia, and remodeling following angioplasty in monkeys with established atherosclerosis. A nonhuman primate model of restenosis. *Arterioscler Thromb Vasc Biol* 16:34-43, 1996.

41. Clowes AW, Reidy MA, Clowes MM: Kinetics of cellular proliferation after arterial injury: I. Smooth muscle growth in the absence of endothelium. *Lab Invest* 49:327-333, 1983.

42. Langille BL, O'Donnell F: Reductions in arterial diameter produced by chronic decreases in blood flow are endothelium-dependent. *Science* 231:405-407, 1986.

43. Zwolak RM, Adams MC, Clowes AW: Kinetics of vein graft hyperplasia: Association with tangential stress. *J Vasc Surg* 5:126-136, 1987.

44. Geary RL, Kohler TR, Vergel S, et al: Time course of flow-induced smooth muscle cell proliferation and intimal thickening in endothelialized baboon vascular grafts. *Circ Res* 74:14-23, 1994.

45. Ferns GA, Raines EW, Sprugel KH, et al: Inhibition of neointimal smooth muscle accumulation after angioplasty by an antibody to PDGF. *Science* 253:1129-1132, 1991.

46. Hanna AK, Fox JC, Neschis DG, et al: Antisense basic fibroblast growth factor gene transfer reduces neointimal thickening after arterial injury. *J Vasc Surg* 25:320-325, 1997.

47. Neschis DG, Safford SD, Hanna AK, et al: Antisense basic fibroblast growth factor gene transfer reduces early intimal thickening in a rabbit femoral artery balloon injury model. *J Vasc Surg* 27:126-134, 1998.
48. Lewis CD, Olson NE, Raines EW, et al: Modulation of smooth muscle proliferation in rat carotid artery by platelet-derived mediators and fibroblast growth factor-2. *Platelets* 12:352-358, 2001.
49. Kim WJ, Chereshnev I, Gazdoiu M, et al: MCP-1 deficiency is associated with reduced intimal hyperplasia after arterial injury. *Biochem Biophys Res Commun* 310:936-942, 2003.
50. Morishita R, Gibbons GH, Ellison KE, et al: Single intraluminal delivery of antisense cdc2 kinase and proliferating-cell nuclear antigen oligonucleotides results in chronic inhibition of neointimal hyperplasia. *Proc Natl Acad Sci U S A* 90:8474-8478, 1993.
51. Mano T, Luo Z, Malendowicz SL, et al: Reversal of GATA-6 downregulation promotes smooth muscle differentiation and inhibits intimal hyperplasia in balloon-injured rat carotid artery. *Circ Res* 84:647-654, 1999.
52. Stephan D, San H, Yang ZY, et al: Inhibition of vascular smooth muscle cell proliferation and intimal hyperplasia by gene transfer of beta-interferon. *Mol Med* 3:593-599, 1997.
53. Chang MW, Ohno T, Gordon D, et al: Adenovirus-mediated transfer of the herpes simplex virus thymidine kinase gene inhibits vascular smooth muscle cell proliferation and neointima formation following balloon angioplasty of the rat carotid artery. *Mol Med* 1:172-181, 1995.
54. Simari RD, San H, Rekhter M, et al: Regulation of cellular proliferation and intimal formation following balloon injury in atherosclerotic rabbit arteries. *J Clin Invest* 98:225-235, 1996.
55. Ueno H, Yamamoto H, Ito S, et al: Adenovirus-mediated transfer of a dominant-negative H-ras suppresses neointimal formation in balloon-injured arteries in vivo. *Arterioscler Thromb Vasc Biol* 17:898-904, 1997.
56. Clowes AW, Clowes MM, Au YP, et al: Smooth muscle cells express urokinase during mitogenesis and tissue-type plasminogen activator during migration in injured rat carotid artery. *Circ Res* 67:61-67, 1990.
57. Nikkari ST, Geary RL, Hatsukami T, et al: Expression of collagen, interstitial collagenase, and tissue inhibitor of metalloproteinases-1 in restenosis after carotid endarterectomy. *Am J Pathol* 148:777-783, 1996.
58. Raper SE, Yudkoff M, Chirmule N, et al: A pilot study of in vivo liver-directed gene transfer with an adenoviral vector in partial ornithine transcarbamylase deficiency. *Hum Gene Ther* 13:163-175, 2002.
59. Raper SE, Grossman M, Rader DJ, et al: Safety and feasibility of liver-directed ex vivo gene therapy for homozygous familial hypercholesterolemia [see comment]. *Ann Surg* 223:116-126, 1996.
60. Sterman DH, Molnar-Kimber K, Iyengar T, et al: A pilot study of systemic corticosteroid administration in conjunction with intrapleural adenoviral vector administration in patients with malignant pleural mesothelioma. *Cancer Gene Ther* 7:1511-1518, 2000.

61. Sterman DH, Treat J, Litzky LA, et al: Adenovirus-mediated herpes simplex virus thymidine kinase/ganciclovir gene therapy in patients with localized malignancy: Results of a phase I clinical trial in malignant mesothelioma. *Hum Gene Ther* 9:1083-1092, 1998.

62. Schulick AH, Vassalli G, Dunn PF, et al: Established immunity precludes adenovirus-mediated gene transfer in rat carotid arteries. Potential for immunosuppression and vector engineering to overcome barriers of immunity. *J Clin Invest* 99:209-219, 1997.

63. Nabel EG, Plautz G, Nabel GJ: Site-specific gene expression in vivo by direct gene transfer into the arterial wall. *Science* 249:1285-1288, 1990.

64. Marshall DJ, Palasis M, Lepore JJ, et al: Biocompatibility of cardiovascular gene delivery catheters with adenovirus vectors: An important determinant of the efficiency of cardiovascular gene transfer. *Mol Ther: J Am Soc Gene Ther* 1:423-429, 2000.

65. Morishita R, Gibbons GH, Kaneda Y, et al: Pharmacokinetics of antisense oligodeoxyribonucleotides (cyclin B1 and CDC 2 kinase) in the vessel wall in vivo: Enhanced therapeutic utility for restenosis by HVJ-liposome delivery. *Gene* 149:13-19, 1994.

66. Zelenock JA, Welling TH, Sarkar R, et al: Improved retroviral transduction efficiency of vascular cells in vitro and in vivo during clinically relevant incubation periods using centrifugation to increase viral titers. *J Vasc Surg* 26:119-127, 1997.

67. Rade JJ, Cheung M, Miyamoto S, et al: Retroviral vector-mediated expression of hirudin by human vascular endothelial cells: Implications for the design of retroviral vectors expressing biologically active proteins. *Gene Ther* 6:385-392, 1999.

68. Geary RL, Clowes AW, Lau S, et al: Gene transfer in baboons using prosthetic vascular grafts seeded with retrovirally transduced smooth muscle cells: A model for local and systemic gene therapy. *Hum Gene Ther* 5:1211-1216, 1994.

69. Wen S, Schneider DB, Driscoll RM, et al: Second-generation adenoviral vectors do not prevent rapid loss of transgene expression and vector DNA from the arterial wall [see comment]. *Arterioscler Thromb Vasc Biol* 20:1452-1458, 2000.

70. Wen S, Driscoll RM, Schneider DB, et al: Inclusion of the E3 region in an adenoviral vector decreases inflammation and neointima formation after arterial gene transfer. *Arterioscler Thromb Vasc Biol* 21:1777-1782, 2001.

71. Newman KD, Dunn PF, Owens JW, et al: Adenovirus-mediated gene transfer into normal rabbit arteries results in prolonged vascular cell activation, inflammation, and neointimal hyperplasia. *J Clin Invest* 96:2955-2965, 1995.

72. Lynch CM, Hara PS, Leonard JC, et al: Adeno-associated virus vectors for vascular gene delivery. *Circ Res* 80:497-505, 1997.

73. Rolling F, Nong Z, Pisvin S, et al: Adeno-associated virus-mediated gene transfer into rat carotid arteries. *Gene Ther* 4:757-761, 1997.

74. Chang DS, Su H, Tang GL, et al: Adeno-associated viral vector-mediated gene transfer of VEGF normalizes skeletal muscle oxygen tension and induces arteriogenesis in ischemic rat hindlimb. *Mol Ther: J Am Soc Gene Ther* 7:44-51, 2003.

75. Curi MA, Skelly CL, Meyerson SL, et al: Sustained inhibition of experimental neointimal hyperplasia with a genetically modified herpes simplex virus. *J Vasc Surg* 37:1294-1300, 2003.

76. Skelly CL, Curi MA, Meyerson SL, et al: Prevention of restenosis by a herpes simplex virus mutant capable of controlled long-term expression in vascular tissue in vivo. *Gene Ther* 8:1840-1846, 2001.

77. Flynn CR, Komalavilas P, Tessier D, et al: Transduction of biologically active motifs of the small heat shock-related protein HSP20 leads to relaxation of vascular smooth muscle. *FASEB J* 17:1358-1360, 2003.

78. Rome JJ, Shayani V, Newman KD, et al: Adenoviral vector-mediated gene transfer into sheep arteries using a double-balloon catheter. *Hum Gene Ther* 5:1249-1258, 1994.

79. Rome JJ, Shayani V, Flugelman MY, et al: Anatomic barriers influence the distribution of in vivo gene transfer into the arterial wall. Modeling with microscopic tracer particles and verification with a recombinant adenoviral vector. *Arterioscl Thromb* 14:148-161, 1994.

80. Naimark WA, Lepore JJ, Klugherz BD, et al: Adenovirus-catheter compatibility increases gene expression after delivery to porcine myocardium. *Hum Gene Ther* 14:161-166, 2003.

81. Nasser TK, Wilensky RL, Mehdi K, et al: Microparticle deposition in periarterial microvasculature and intramural dissections after porous balloon delivery into atherosclerotic vessels: Quantitation and localization by confocal scanning laser microscopy. *Am Heart J* 131:892-898, 1996.

82. Wilensky RL, March KL, Gradus-Pizlo I, et al: Regional and arterial localization of radioactive microparticles after local delivery by unsupported or supported porous balloon catheters. *Am Heart J* 129:852-859, 1995.

83. Simons M, Edelman ER, DeKeyser JL, et al: Antisense c-myb oligonucleotides inhibit intimal arterial smooth muscle cell accumulation in vivo. *Nature* 359:67-70, 1992.

84. Lombardi JV, Naji M, Larson RA, et al: Adenoviral mediated uteroglobin gene transfer to the adventitia reduces arterial intimal hyperplasia. *J Surg Res* 99:377-380, 2001.

85. Conte MS, Birinyi LK, Miyata T, et al: Efficient repopulation of denuded rabbit arteries with autologous genetically modified endothelial cells. *Circulation* 89:2161-2169, 1994.

86. Fortuin FD, Vale P, Losordo DW, et al: One-year follow-up of direct myocardial gene transfer of vascular endothelial growth factor-2 using naked plasmid deoxyribonucleic acid by way of thoracotomy in no-option patients. *Am J Cardiol* 92:436-439, 2003.

87. Vale PR, Isner JM, Rosenfield K: Therapeutic angiogenesis in critical limb and myocardial ischemia. *J Intervent Cardiol* 14:511-528, 2001.

88. Mohler ER 3rd, Rajagopalan S, Olin JW, et al: Adenoviral-mediated gene transfer of vascular endothelial growth factor in critical limb ischemia: Safety results from a phase I trial. *Vasc Med* 8:9-13, 2003.

89. Ehsan A, Mann MJ, Dell'Acqua G, et al: Long-term stabilization of vein graft wall architecture and prolonged resistance to experimental atherosclerosis after E2F decoy oligonucleotide gene therapy. *J Thorac Cardiovasc Surg* 121:714-722, 2001.

90. von der Leyen HE, Braun-Dullaeus R, Mann MJ, et al: A pressure-mediated nonviral method for efficient arterial gene and oligonucleotide transfer. *Hum Gene Ther* 10:2355-2364, 1999.

91. Morishita R, Gibbons GH, Horiuchi M, et al: A gene therapy strategy using a transcription factor decoy of the E2F binding site inhibits smooth muscle proliferation in vivo. *Proc Natl Acad Sci U S A* 92:5855-5859, 1995.

92. Mann MJ, Whittemore AD, Donaldson MC, et al: Ex-vivo gene therapy of human vascular bypass grafts with E2F decoy: The PREVENT single-centre, randomised, controlled trial. *Lancet* 354:1493-1498, 1999.

93. Grube E: Phase II trial of the E2F decoy in coronary bypass grafting. *Circulation* 2001.

94. Tzeng E, Shears LL, Robbins PD, et al: Vascular gene transfer of the human inducible nitric oxide synthase: Characterization of activity and effects on myointimal hyperplasia. *Mol Med* 2:211-225, 1996.

95. Kibbe MR, Tzeng E, Gleixner SL, et al: Adenovirus-mediated gene transfer of human inducible nitric oxide synthase in porcine vein grafts inhibits intimal hyperplasia. *J Vasc Surg* 34:156-165, 2001.

96. Shears LL, Kibbe MR, Murdock AD, et al: Efficient inhibition of intimal hyperplasia by adenovirus-mediated inducible nitric oxide synthase gene transfer to rats and pigs in vivo. *J Am Coll Surg* 187:295-306, 1998.

CHAPTER 9

Angiogenesis in Limb Ischemia

Albeir Y. Mousa, MD
Vascular Research Fellow, Division of Vascular Surgery, New York–Presbyterian Hospital, Weill Medical College of Cornell University, Columbia University College of Physicians & Surgeons, New York, NY

Peter Henderson, BA
Vascular Research Fellow, Division of Vascular Surgery, New York–Presbyterian Hospital, Weill Medical College of Cornell University, Columbia University College of Physicians & Surgeons, New York, NY

K. Craig Kent, MD, FACS
Professor of Surgery, Chief, Division of Vascular Surgery, New York–Presbyterian Hospital, Weill Medical College of Cornell University, Columbia University College of Physicians & Surgeons, New York, NY

Circulatory impairment is a major cause of morbidity and mortality in the United States. More than 200,000 persons develop symptoms of lower extremity ischemia each year, and it is estimated that 150,000 patients per year require lower limb amputation because of ischemic peripheral vascular disease. Atherosclerosis is the most common cause. Although patients with atherosclerotic occlusions develop collateral circulation, collateral networks are never sufficient to completely restore the deficiency in circulation produced by a major arterial occlusion.

Revascularization remains the mainstay of therapy for lower extremity ischemia. Both catheter-based interventions and surgical bypass have been extremely effective in reducing the morbidity associated with this disease process. However, not all patients with peripheral arterial disease are candidates for intervention. In some patients, severe distal disease precludes operative intervention, as can be the case in patients with diabetes, renal insufficiency, or Buerger disease. In still other patients, multiple comorbidities associated with cardiac or cerebrovascular disease preclude the use of invasive treatments. Consequently, a less invasive strategy would be a welcome adjunct to the current therapeutic alternatives for patients with lower extremity occlusive disease.

One proposed alternative is therapeutic angiogenesis. Therapeutic angiogenesis is defined as the use of a biological active agent or device to stimulate the formation of new blood vessels in ischemic tissues. Administration of angiogenic proteins to reestablish blood flow in an ischemic extremity could potentially allow the creation of an endogenous or biological "bypass."

There are 2 potential mechanisms that can lead to the growth of new blood vessels. The first is through sprouting of new capillaries (classic angiogenesis). The second is through the growth of new arterioles (arteriogenesis). These dynamic processes are mediated by proteins known as growth factors and their cellular receptors located within ischemic tissues. Studies in animals have repeatedly proven that the exogenous administration of a variety of growth factors, particularly fibroblast growth factor (FGF) and vascular endothelial growth factor (VEGF), can augment blood flow in regions of arterial ischemia and improve tissue perfusion. The clinical application of these techniques, however, is in its infancy. In this chapter, the current "state of the art" of therapeutic angiogenesis for peripheral vascular disease is reviewed.

ANGIOGENIC GROWTH FACTORS

A variety of growth factors and cytokines have been shown to have angiogenic properties. At least 20 growth factors are known to stimulate angiogenesis, and a number of these have been evaluated in clinical trials of angiogenesis. Although all of these proteins are similar in that they can initiate or propagate the angiogenic or arteriogenic process, there are notable differences in their behavior and function. Ultimately, therapeutic angiogenesis may be best produced by using a combination of these various angiogenic proteins.

VEGF

VEGF is a family of 34- to 46-kd dimeric glycoproteins with 8 exons found on chromosome 6 at 6p21.3. These proteins were initially characterized as vascular permeability factors, although in 1989 VEGF was cloned as an angiogenic factor.[1] Splicing of the VEGF-A gene results in 5 isoforms ($VEGF_{121}$, $VEGF_{145}$, $VEGF_{165}$, $VEGF_{189}$, $VEGF_{206}$) differing in the total number of amino acids.[2] It is probable that these isoforms have different functions in the angiogenic process. Most cell types produce several VEGF isoforms; however, the most commonly expressed proteins are $VEGF_{121}$ and $VEGF_{165}$. VEGF has a signaling sequence that permits its secretion by intact cells. Thus, VEGF produced in transfected cells has the ability to be secreted and become immediately biologically active. VEGF appears to be the most potent regulator of angiogenesis.[3] Loss of even one VEGF allele results in embryonic lethality. Although VEGF is synthesized by a variety of cell types in and around the vessel wall, this protein specifically affects endothelial cell proliferation and migration by binding to 2 transmembrane tyrosine kinase receptors.[4] Moreover, VEGF enhances endothelial cell survival, an event that complements its mitogenic effect. Although VEGF does not have a direct effect on smooth muscle cells or pericytes, indirectly, through factors released by endothelial cells, VEGF can stimulate smooth muscle cell migration and proliferation. Hypoxia is a potent stimulus for VEGF expression.[5] Transcription of VEGF messenger RNA (mRNA) is mediated in part by the binding of hypoxia-inducible factor 1 to a binding site located on the VEGF promoter.[6] Furthermore, VEGF mRNA is intrinsically labile; however, in response to hypoxia, there is stabilization of its mRNA.[7,8] VEGF also increases expression of plasminogen activator and collagenase in endothelial cells, which in turn, degrade extracellular matrix, allowing endothelial cell migration and sprouting. Thus, VEGF plays a number of distinct roles in the angiogenic process.

FGF

FGF is a family of structurally homologous 16- to 24-kd proteins that enhance proliferation of endothelial cells, fibroblasts, and smooth muscle cells. At present, the FGF family is known to include at least 20 different proteins.[9] Unlike VEGF, the classic FGFs, FGF-1 and FGF-2 (also known as acidic and basic FGF, respectively), lack the signal sequence that allows their direct cellular secretion.[10] Thus, genetic techniques used to express FGF must be accompanied by a mechanism that facilitates protein secretion. FGF has no effect on vascular permeability. The biological effects of FGFs are mediated by 4 structurally related tyrosine kinase receptors, which are broadly expressed.[11,12]

Like VEGF, FGF stimulates angiogenesis and collateral vessel formation. FGF, however, also directly stimulates smooth muscle cell proliferation, which can lead to intimal thickening and blood vessel occlusion. FGF also regulates the expression of several additional molecules that are critical to angiogenesis, such as interstitial collagenase, urokinase-type plasminogen activator, plasminogen activator inhibitor-1, the urokinase-type plasminogen activator receptor, and β1 integrins. Thus, administration of FGF can have both beneficial and adverse effects on the vascular system. Moreover, systemic treatment with FGF has been associated with renal and hematologic toxicity, both of which may affect the potential therapeutic use of this protein.[13]

HEPATOCYTE GROWTH FACTOR/SCATTER FACTOR

Recent studies have identified the protein hepatocyte growth factor (HGF) as an angiogenic growth factor. First discovered in the late 1980s, it is also known as scatter factor and shows homology to the enzymes of the blood coagulation cascade. HGF is synthesized as a biologically inactive single-chain precursor weighing 83 kd that is cleaved by a specific extracellular serum serine protease to a fully active heterodimer composed of the 2 disulfide-linked cleavage products. It is a mesenchyme-derived factor that regulates growth, motility, and morphogenesis of various cell types, most importantly endothelial cells.[14,15] It is known to be crucial to development, as knockout mice display an embryonic lethal phenotype. HGF is similar to VEGF in that it contains a sequence that allows secretion of the protein from cells.

TISSUE HYPOXIA AND TISSUE HYPOXIA FACTOR

Tissue hypoxia is an extremely important physiologic stimulus of endogenous angiogenesis. Hypoxia appears to be the stimulant for the angiogenesis that accompanies wound healing as well as lower extremity vascular insufficiency. The effects of hypoxia are in large part mediated by hypoxia-inducible factor-1 (HIF-1), which is a heterodimeric transcription factor that regulates the expression of a number of oxygen-dependent genes, including VEGF. The VEGF gene contains a hypoxia response element within its promoter that is responsive to this factor.[12] Thus, as a novel approach, gene transfer of HIF-1 might be used to stimulate angiogenesis. Although HIF-1 has been used in animal models with some success, to date, clinical trials of HIF-1 have not been initiated.

METHODS OF DELIVERY FOR ANGIOGENIC PROTEINS

Although angiogenic growth factors have been demonstrated to enhance collateral vessel formation, of critical importance is the technique for delivery of these agents to ischemic tissues. There are 2 major methods of delivery. Protein can be directly injected into tissues. The advantage of this approach is that proteins are bioactive and can directly stimulate angiogenesis. The half-life of these proteins, however, is relatively short, and a sustained effect is difficult to achieve without repeated treatments. Nevertheless, direct administration of proteins has been used in a number of clinical trials of therapeutic angiogenesis.

Alternatively, gene therapy or gene transfer results in a "turned-on" gene that leads to the continuous release of high concentrations of therapeutic protein over a sustained period. For gene transfer to be successful, however, the foreign gene must cross the outer membrane of the host cell. To accomplish this, the gene is first inserted into a plasmid, a naturally occurring circular DNA molecule. The plasmid (or naked DNA) can be directly applied to tissues. Since the uptake of naked DNA by cells is limited, high concentrations of naked DNA are required, and expression of the transfected gene is often weak. Alternatively, a carrier, referred to as a vector, can be used to deliver recombinant DNA into a host cell. Viruses are commonly used vectors. Transfection efficiencies can be achieved with adenoviruses that are many times greater than what can be achieved by exposing cells to naked DNA.[16] Unfortunately, when an adenovirus is used to infect a target cell, a host immune response is incited against the adenovirus. Neutralizing antibodies to the adenovirus then form, and these antibodies limit the duration of DNA expression[17] and also eliminate the possibility of using an adenoviral vector on subsequent occasions.[18] Thus, the advantage of naked DNA is that it can be injected on multiple occasions (but transfection efficiencies and protein production may be low). Alternatively, the advantage of adenoviral vectors is that high levels of genetic expression and protein production can be achieved (but immune responses limit the durability of the effect). The optimal approach to therapeutic angiogenesis is yet to be determined and may vary with the growth factor or the tissue being treated.

Regardless of the form of delivery, angiogenic proteins can be introduced into ischemic tissues via 2 different techniques. Genes can be injected directly into the arterial circulation proximal to an occlusion. This approach allows the genetic material to be dispersed into collaterals and presumably carried distally to the point where neovascularization might be optimally needed. Systemic toxicity is a potential side effect of this approach. Local delivery can be achieved by direct injection of the angiogenic protein into the muscles through which collaterals pass. Local injection markedly diminishes the potential for systemic toxicity and confines the expression of the protein to the tissues into which the gene has been injected.[19,20] Both approaches have been used in clinical trials of angiogenesis.

CLINICAL TRIALS

Innumerable preclinical studies in animals have established that angiogenic growth factors can promote collateral and capillary development in models of peripheral and myocardial ischemia. Human clinical experience with therapeutic angiogenesis for the treatment of myocardial and lower extremity ischemia is gradually accumulating, with several trials under way. The results of these trials have been mixed. Some have demonstrated little or no clinical benefit, whereas the outcome of others has been encouraging. Outlined below are results from completed or ongoing clinical trials of therapeutic angiogenesis for peripheral vascular disease.

VEGF TRIALS

In the first significant trial of therapeutic angiogenesis for peripheral vascular disease, Baumgartner et al[21] in 1998 reported the results of a phase I clinical trial of intramuscular injection of $VEGF_{165}$ in 9 patients with critical limb ischemia. The majority of these patients had either rest pain or a nonhealing ulcer, and all were not considered candidates for surgical or percutaneous revascularization. Gene transfer was performed by intramuscular injection of 2000 µg of naked plasmid DNA encoding $VEGF_{165}$ into the calves and thighs of symptomatic patients. These injections were performed on 2 occasions separated by a 4-week interval. Successful gene expression in patients was documented by an increase in serum VEGF levels. Angiography and magnetic resonance angiography were performed prior and 4 weeks after these treatments, and patients were followed up for an average of 6 months. The investigators noted a significant improvement in the average ankle-brachial index (ABI) at 12 weeks, from 0.33 to 0.48. Contrast angiography was thought to demonstrate new collateral vessels in 7 limbs, and magnetic resonance angiography revealed improved distal flow in 8 limbs. There was resolution in all 3 patients who presented with solitary rest pain. Four of 7 ischemic ulcers either healed or improved. Only 3 of the 9 patients subsequently required below-knee amputation.

In an additional study, 6 patients with Buerger disease and critical limb ischemia were treated by the same investigators.[22] These patients were treated twice at 4-week intervals, with 2 or 4 mg of intramuscular $VEGF_{165}$. New collateral formation was evident in all 7 limbs as demonstrated by magnetic resonance angiography and contrast angiography. Healing of gangrenous ulcers or toes occurred in 3 patients. Nocturnal rest pain was relieved in 2 patients. Two patients with pre-established necrotic lesions of the forefoot eventually required amputation.

The value of VEGF gene therapy in the treatment of peripheral neuropathy has been evaluated in patients with critical limb ischemia. Twenty-nine patients received intramuscular injections of plasmid $VEGF_{165}$ human plasmid.[23] Evaluations were performed before and after treatment and included an assessment of symptoms, a clinical examination, and electrophysiologic studies. Seventeen patients (19 limbs) completed the 6-month study. Compared with baseline, treated patients had a significant increase in symptom and clinical scores and in the electrophysiologic studies. Improvement in ABI in treated legs corresponded to an improvement in neuropathy. Neurologic improvement was seen in 4 of the 6 patients with diabetes who completed the study, demonstrating that the presence of diabetes did not preclude a response to therapy. The authors of this study concluded that, as demonstrated in this preliminary evaluation, VEGF can reverse the symptoms and findings of neuropathy in ischemic limbs.

In 2003, Rajagopalan et al[24] reported the results of the Regional Angiogenesis with Vascular Endothelial Growth Factor (RAVE) trial. Notably, this was the first randomized trial using VEGF for angiogenesis. In this phase II, double-blind, placebo-controlled evaluation, the efficacy of intramuscular injection of adenoviral $VEGF_{121}$ in patients with critical limb ischemia was evaluated. A total of 105 patients were randomly assigned to 1 of 3 groups: low-dose VEGF (4 × 10^9 particle units), high-dose VEGF (4 × 10^{10} particle units), or placebo. Efficacy was evaluated by using the outcome measure of peak walking time, ABI, claudication distance, and quality of life. Unfortunately, there was no demonstrable improvement in either exercise performance or quality of life in the patients treated.

FIBROBLAST GROWTH FACTOR (FGF) TRIALS

Lazarous et al[25] initiated a double-blind, placebo-controlled, dose-escalation trial in patients with claudication who had an ABI of less than 0.8. Patients were randomly assigned to placebo (n = 6), 10 µg/kg of bFGF (n = 4), 30 µg/kg of bFGF once (n = 5), and 30 µg/kg of bFGF on 2 consecutive days (n = 4). FGF was infused into the femoral artery of ischemic legs. The half-life of FGF in the circulation was approximately 46 minutes. Calf blood flow, which was measured by strain gauge plethysmography, increased at 1 month by 66% ± 26% (mean ± SEM) and at 6 months by 153% ± 51% in bFGF-treated patients (n = 9, $P = .002$). The investigators concluded that bFGF was well tolerated by patients, although demonstration of efficacy required further evaluation.

In a recently completed phase II, multicenter, randomized, double-blind, placebo-controlled trial (TRAFFIC, Chiron Corp),[26] patients with intermittent claudication were randomly assigned to receive placebo or 1 or 2 doses of recombinant FGF-2 protein (30 µg/kg) provided intra-arterially on day 1 or days 1 and 30. A total of 192 patients were enrolled. Patients were included if they had symptomatic claudication with a resting ABI of less than 0.8. Outcome measures included a change in peak walking time and quality of life at 90 and 180 days. The results demonstrated a statistically significant increase in peak walking time at 90 days in the single-dose cohort but not in the double-dose group. At 180 days, treatment with FGF did not alter the peak walking time, claudication severity, stair climbing, walking speed, or walking distance. Despite the single isolated positive finding at 90 days, the results of this trial, in general, were discouraging, and further investigation with this technique has not been undertaken.

In another multicenter trial, the gene for FGF-1 was used to treat patients with limb-threatening lower extremity ischemia.[27] A total of 51 patients with unreconstructible end-stage lower limb ischemia underwent treatment with intramuscular injection of the FGF plasmid. In a trial that was designed primarily for safety, patients were injected into the thigh and calf with repeated and escalating concentrations of plasmid FGF (500, 1000, 2000, 4000, 8000, and 16,000 µg). This was not a randomized trial; thus, comparison with placebo was not made. Outcome measures included serum levels of FGF, transcutaneous oxygen pressure, ABI, pain, and ulcer healing in the ischemic extremity. A significant reduction in pain and aggregate ulcer size was associated with an increased transcutaneous oxygen pressure compared with baseline pretreatment values. Also, a significant increase in ABI was observed. Arteriograms performed before and after treatment demonstrated evidence of new blood vessel growth. The authors of this study concluded that FGF might be effective in the treatment of patients with end-stage lower extremity vascular disease. Further validation of this hypothesis awaits the results of a randomized, placebo-controlled trial that is currently under way.

HGF TRIALS

There is an ongoing clinical trial sponsored by AnGes and Daiichi Pharmaceuticals to study the safety and efficacy of HGF via plasmid vector (AMG0001) in the treatment of patients with critical limb ischemia. This phase II, randomized, double-blind, placebo-controlled study is designed to enroll 100 patients and evaluate the ability of AMG0001 to produce a reduction in amputation, rest pain, and mortality, as well as an increase in wound healing and improvement in patients' quality of life. Results of this trial may be forthcoming within the next 2 years.

STEM CELLS

Recently, autologous bone marrow has been explored as a technique for stimulating angiogenesis. Contained within bone marrow are endothelial progenitor cells, which have the capacity to differentiate into capillaries and arterioles. Endothelial progenitor cells in embryonic tissues are the precursors to new blood vessels.[28] Moreover, Asahara et al[29] have shown that endothelial progenitor cells circulate in adult peripheral blood. In addition, endothelial progenitor cells secrete various angiogenic growth factors and cytokines, which in turn potentiate the angiogenic process. In a randomized, double-blind, placebo-controlled trial, researchers in Japan injected autologous bone marrow into the ischemic extremities of 47 patients with intermittent claudication. These investigators found improvement in a number of outcome measures, including an increase in ABI and pain-free walking time. These results were maintained for up to 24 weeks.[30] Although biologically modified endothelial progenitor cells may be a potent therapeutic alternative for enhancing angiogenesis, validation of this awaits larger and randomized trials that are currently under way.

ANGIOGENIC THERAPY: COMPLICATIONS

There are potential drawbacks to the use of growth factors and angiogenic agents in the treatment of lower extremity occlusive disease. VEGF is a vascular permeability factor and can potentially produce edema in the treated extremity. Angiogenic agents also carry the risk of stimulating neovascularization in nontarget tissues such as the eyes or joints. Because tumor growth is dependent on angiogenesis, there is potential risk with administration of angiogenic factors of accelerating the progression of latent tumors. Angiogenic factors may also cause unnatural cellular proliferation leading to the initial development of malignant lesions. There is also concern that VEGF and other growth factors could lead to progression of atherosclerosis as well as plaque instability and rupture. The actual risk of any of these untoward events is unknown. Fortunately, most normal tissues do not express measurable levels of the receptors for many of these proteins. To date, none of these effects have been observed in animals or in human clinical trials.

FUTURE INVESTIGATION

The mixed outcomes of current human trials involving angiogenesis may be related to a variety of factors. Progress has been slow in refining methods of gene transfer. Needed are improvements in the durability, efficacy, and specificity of gene expression. The emergence of novel, safe, and more effective vectors will improve the feasibility of therapeutic angiogenesis. It is now widely recognized that both angiogenesis and arteriogenesis require the cooperative action of multiple cytokines and growth factors. Thus, gene therapy with combinations of vectors/plasmids (gene cocktails) may offer another strategy that increases overall efficacy. It has recently been discovered that nitric oxide (NO) is critical to the success of angiogenic therapy. NO appears to be important in arteriogenesis and leads to early dilatation of small collateral vessels. Thus, strategies to stimulate the production of NO may be yet another method of enhancing blood flow to ischemic tissues. Angiotensin-converting enzyme (ACE) inhibitors are another powerful class of medications with significant effects on endothelial function. ACE inhibitors block the generation of angiotensin II and prevent the breakdown of bradykinin, an important mediator of NO release. ACE inhibitors improve endothelial dysfunction in patients with coronary disease and have been shown to stimulate angiogenesis and collateral vessel formation in a rabbit ischemic hindlimb model.[31]

SUMMARY

Clinical studies of therapeutic angiogenesis in humans are at a very early stage, and the preliminary results are inconclusive. Many of the early trials have been phase I investigations testing safety rather than efficacy. As such, patients in these trials have received only the experimental therapy. Since it is well established that some patients with severe peripheral vascular disease can, with proper treatment, heal their wounds and have resolution of rest pain, positive findings in nonrandomized trials must be interpreted with caution. Patients with lower extremity occlusive disease manifesting as claudication or limb-threatening ischemia are a heterogeneous group. In this patient population, experience with other treatment modalities has demonstrated that efficacy can only be proven through large randomized trials.

There is still much to learn about the complex processes of angiogenesis and arteriogenesis. Phase I trials with new agents, combination therapy, and stem cells are under way at many institutions, including our own. The promise of this technique is great. It is possible that advances over the next several years will transform therapeutic angiogenesis from a novel concept to a practical treatment for lower extremity vascular insufficiency.

REFERENCES

1. Ferrara N, Henzel WJ: Pituitary follicular cells secrete a novel heparin-binding growth factor specific for vascular endothelial cells. *Biochem Biophys Res Commun* 161:851-858, 1989.
2. Ferrara N: Vascular endothelial growth factor: Molecular and biological aspects. *Curr Top Microbiol Immunol* 237:1-30, 1999.
3. Rissanen TT, Markkanen JE, Gruchala M, et al: VEGF-D is the strongest angiogenic and lymphangiogenic effector among VEGFs delivered into skeletal muscle via adenoviruses. *Circ Res* 92:1098-1106, 2003.
4. Shibuya M, Ito N, Claesson-Welsh L: Structure and function of vascular endothelial growth factor receptor-1 and -2. *Curr Top Microbiol Immunol* 237:59-83, 1999.
5. Levy AP, Levy NS, Wegner S, et al: Transcriptional regulation of the rat vascular endothelial growth factor gene by hypoxia. *J Biol Chem* 270:13333-13340, 1995.
6. Semenza GL: HIF-1, O (2), and the 3 PHDs: How animal cells signal hypoxia to the nucleus. *Cell* 107:1-3, 2001.
7. Ross J: mRNA stability in mammalian cells. *Microbiol Rev* 59:423-450, 1995.
8. Paulding WR, Czyzyk-Krzeska MF: Hypoxia-induced regulation of mRNA stability. *Adv Exp Med Biol* 475:111-121, 2000.
9. Jaye M, Schlessinger J, Dionne CA: Fibroblast growth factor receptor tyrosine kinases: Molecular analysis and signal transduction. *Biochim Biophys Acta* 1135:185-199, 1992.
10. Szebenyi G, Fallon JF: Fibroblast growth factors as multifunctional signaling factors. *Int Rev Cytol* 185:45-106, 1999.
11. Unger EF, Epstein SE, Chew EY, et al: Effects of a single intracoronary injection of basic fibroblast growth factor in stable angina pectoris. *Am J Cardiol* 85:1414-1419, 2000.
12. Semenza GL: Hypoxia inducible factor 1: Master regulator of oxygen homeostasis. *Curr Opin Genet Dev* 8:588-594, 1999.
13. Unger EF, Goncalves L, Epstein SE, et al: Effects of a single intracoronary injection of basic fibroblast growth factor in stable angina pectoris. *Am J Cardiol* 85:1414-1419, 2000.
14. Matsumoto K, Nakamura T: Emerging multipotent aspects of hepatocyte growth factor. *J Biochem (Tokyo)* 119:591-600, 1996.
15. Matsumoto K, Nakamura T: Hepatocyte growth factor (HGF) as tissue organizer for organogenesis and regeneration. *Biochem Biophys Res Commun* 239:639-644, 1997.
16. Nabel EG, Nabel GJ: Complex models for the study of gene function in cardiovascular biology. *Annu Rev Physiol* 56:741-761, 1994.

17. Wilson JM: Adenoviruses as gene-delivery vehicles. *N Engl J Med* 334: 1185-1187, 1996.
18. Zabner J, Petersen DM, Puga AP, et al: Safety and efficacy of repetitive adenovirus-mediated transfer of CFTR cDNA to airway epithelia of primates and cotton rats. *Nat Genet* 6:75-83, 1994.
19. Wolff JA, Malone RW, Williams P, et al: Direct gene transfer into mouse muscle in vivo. *Science* 247:1465-1468, 1990.
20. Lin H, Parmacek MS, Morle G, et al: Expression of recombinant genes in myocardium in vivo after direct injection of DNA. *Circulation* 82:2217-2221, 1990.
21. Baumgartner I, Pieczek A, Manor O, et al: Constitutive expression of phVEGF165 after intramuscular gene transfer promotes collateral vessel development in patients with critical limb ischemia. *Circulation* 97: 1114-1123, 1998.
22. Isner JM, Baumgartner I, Rauh G, et al: Treatment of thromboangiitis obliterans (Buerger's disease) by intramuscular gene transfer of vascular endothelial growth factor: Preliminary clinical results. *J Vasc Surg* 28:964-973, 1998.
23. Simovic D, Isner JM, Ropper AH, et al: Improvement in chronic ischemic neuropathy after intramuscular phVEGF165 gene transfer in patients with critical limb ischemia. *Arch Neurol* 58:761-768, 2001.
24. Rajagopalan S, Mohler ER III, Lederman RJ: Regional angiogenesis with vascular endothelial growth factor in peripheral arterial disease: A phase II randomized, double-blind, controlled study of adenoviral delivery of vascular endothelial growth factor 121 in patients with disabling intermittent claudication. *Circulation* 108:1933-1938, 2003.
25. Lazarous DF, Unger EF, Epstein SE, et al: Basic fibroblast growth factor in patients with intermittent claudication: Results of a phase I trial. *J Am Coll Cardiol* 36:1239-1244, 2000.
26. Lederman RJ, Mendelsohn FO, Anderson RD: Therapeutic angiogenesis with recombinant fibroblast growth factor-2 for intermittent claudication (the TRAFFIC study): A randomised trial. *Lancet* 359:2053-2058, 2002.
27. Comerota AJ, Throm RC, Miller KA: Naked plasmid DNA encoding fibroblast growth factor type 1 for the treatment of end-stage unreconstructible lower extremity ischemia: Preliminary results of a phase I trials. *J Vasc Surg* 35:930-936, 2002.
28. Asahara T, Masuda H, Takahashi T, et al: Bone marrow origin of endothelial progenitor cells responsible for postnatal vasculogenesis in physiological and pathological neovascularization. *Circ Res* 85:221-228, 1999.
29. Asahara T, Murohara T, Sullivan A, et al: Isolation of putative progenitor endothelial cells for angiogenesis. *Science* 275:964-967, 1997.
30. Tateishi-Yuyama E, Matsubara H, Murohara T: Therapeutic angiogenesis for patients with limb ischaemia by autologous transplantation of

bone-marrow cells: A pilot study and a randomised controlled trial. *Lancet* 360:427-435, 2002.

31. Fabre JE, Rivard A, Magner M, et al: Tissue inhibition of angiotensin-converting enzyme activity stimulates angiogenesis in vivo. *Circulation* 99:3043-3049, 1999.

CHAPTER 10

New Advances in the Treatment of Wounds

John C. Lantis II, MD
Assistant Professor of Surgery, Columbia University College of
Physicians and Surgeons, Assistant Attending in Surgery, New York
Presbyterian Hospital, New York, NY

Chronic wound care has come a long way over the last 20 years. The wound care industry is constantly turning out new products, with approximately 3000 products currently available in the United States. Chronic wounds are traditionally defined as "those wounds that fail to progress through an orderly and timely sequence of repair or wounds that pass through the repair process without restoring anatomic and functional results."[1] Histologically, chronic wounds have been observed to differ from acute wounds in a number of ways.[2] The most common chronic wounds include lower extremity diabetic ulcers, venous stasis ulcers, and ischemic ulcers. For a variety of reasons, the stages of wound healing—the vascular response, blood coagulation, inflammation, neovascularization, granulation, fibrinolysis, contraction, epithelialization, and scar formation—are blunted or inhibited. A thickened epidermal border, a fibrotic cuff, and significant extracellular matrix at the base are associated with chronic wounds. These result in a prolonged period of failed reepithelialization and continued inflammation fueled by an excess of proinflammatory cytokines, eventually leading to delayed healing and persistence of granulation tissue in the wound bed.[3]

WHY WOUNDS DO NOT HEAL: WOUND BED PREPARATION

An increasing awareness of the problem of chronic wound healing and society's increased interest in wounds because of the huge health care burden they impose have led to many advances over the last 40 years. The first of these advancements is embodied by the concept of moist wound healing. In 1962, Winter[4] showed that wounds reepithelialize more rapidly under moist conditions. Since that time, there has been ongoing development of a variety of dressings that facilitate the maintenance of a moist wound environment. A large body of literature has developed around the concept of wound bed preparation, which focuses on optimizing the microenvironment of chronic wounds.[5] It is becoming clear that our most advanced chronic wound care closure algorithms will not work unless the correct host environment is achieved.

Wound debridement alone does not constitute adequate wound bed preparation. The concept has been that wound debridement is an effective way to remove necrotic tissue and bacteria, which should be the only impediments to wound healing. Therefore, all wounds should heal after debridement! In chronic wounds, however, many additional factors need to be addressed. Chronic wounds have what is known as the "necrotic burden," which consists of both necrotic tissue and exudate.[5] This necrotic exudate contains matrix metalloproteases (MMPs) that act to break down extracellular matrix proteins and delay wound healing.[6-8] Falanga[9] outlines a continuum of basic to complex abnormalities in wound healing that range from edema and the presence of necrotic tissue to corrupt matrix and phenotypic changes in resident cells. The treatment of these factors ranges from the mundane to the esoteric, with considerable overlap among the corrective measures. It may seem as if the easiest way to correct the various abnormalities of chronic wound healing is to excise the wound and turn it into an acute wound. Unfortunately, this does not always remove all the host and confounding variables that led to delayed healing in the first place. In general, this simply places an acute wound in a "chronic wound environment." However, it should be noted that the acute injury response may occasionally be beneficial in the senescent environment.

Wound bed preparation includes the removal of necrotic and fibrinous tissue, control of edema, maintenance or achievement of a well-vascularized wound bed, control of bacterial burden, and minimization of the wound exudate. Addressing these various issues starts with a thorough evaluation of the host, followed by the application of modern and sometimes novel wound care healing algorithms. The 3 pillars to chronic wound care include (1) addressing the cause of delayed wound healing, (2) providing appropriate local wound care, and (3) addressing the concerns of the patient.[10]

IMPORTANCE OF MOISTURE IN WOUND CARE

In 1958, Odland noted that the wound underneath a blister healed faster when the blister was kept intact. This is probably the first observation of the importance of moisture in wound healing.[11] Winter[4] subsequently noted that the rate of epithelialization in a pig wound when covered with polyethylene films was double that of wounds healing under a dry scab. Stemming from this work is a large body of evidence that supports the concept that moist is superior to dry wound care. In a moist wound environment, the production of collagen is increased significantly in the wound bed.[12] In contrast, wounds exposed to air are more fibroplastic, fibrotic, and scarred.[12] Occlusive dressings maintain a normal voltage gradient across the wound, whereas dry wounds are devoid of an electrical gradient.[13] This electrical gradient may be important for epidermal cell migration.[13-15] It has been postulated that in a dry environment, epidermal cells are inhibited from migrating and providing coverage of the wound because they are forced to migrate between the eschar and the underlying living tissue, whereas in the moist wound, reepithelialization occurs more rapidly because of the absence of crust formation.

No therapy, however, is without its potential drawbacks. Moist environments can lead to maceration of the surrounding skin. This is especially true in wounds with heavy exudate. In wounds dressed in an occlusive fashion, this can occur if the dressing does not allow for the passage of water vapor. Therefore, a dressing should be chosen that allows for just enough moisture to obtain the benefits of accelerated healing but prevent the accumulation of significant fluid between the dressing and the wound.[15] Besides the benefits of more rapid epidermal migration, increased collagen deposition, and decreased fibrosis, the moist wound environment allows for autolytic debridement. This is the process by which autologous enzymes are allowed to debride nonviable tissue. Moisture-retentive dressings trap leukocytes as they collect in the wound exudates, and as these cells die, they release their lysosomal enzymes, which act to degrade proteins and mucopolysaccharides. Since bacteria can also be trapped under these dressings, changing the dressing at the appropriate interval can prevent the bacterial burden from becoming too high. Although the surfaces of most wounds are colonized by both aerobes and anaerobes, occlusive dressings have been shown to keep out harmful organisms.[16] Hutchinson has documented that occlusive dressings produce a lower incidence of infection than open-air or gauze dressings. Traditional gauze and wet to dry dressings tend to stick to wounds, and their removal can disrupt the wound bed and actually lead to a delay in wound healing, whereas in the moist wound environment, the dressing has minimal contact with the newly forming dermis. This moist environment further enhances wound healing by preventing tissue dehydration and cell death, and by promoting release of growth factors that promote angiogenesis.[17]

FORMULARY

The modern wound care formulary boasts a confusing 2400+ products that are made by a variety of companies too numerous to catalog. It is important that the clinician know the basic differences between the various categories of wound care products. All purport to facilitate moist wound care and wound bed preparation. These products include hydrogels, hydrocolloids, foam dressings, alginates, enzymatic debriders, and antimicrobial dressings. Practitioners should be familiar with at least one product in each category so that they can command the full armamentarium of resources that have the potential to enhance wound care.

HYDROGELS

These dressings offer the first line in moist wound care. They are hydrophilic and nonadherent polymers that contain a large percentage of water and actually can absorb up to 5 times their own weight in water. They maintain the wound's moist environment by attracting water molecules to the hydrophilic polysaccharide particles that make up a portion of the polymer. They do not adhere to the wound and provide a cooling and soothing effect. In addition, they hydrate eschar and allow for autolytic debridement. The gels can be delivered in many forms including amorphous gels, sheets, and strands. They are usually left in place for 24 hours and washed off the wound. This type of dressing is appropriate for wounds with mild exudates, clean wounds, and partial-thickness wounds. Commercially available products in this category include Solosite, Purilon, Woun'Dres, Nu-Gel, Duoderm gel, Flexigel, Carrasyn gel, Curasol, and Curafil gel, among others.

HYDROCOLLOIDS

Hydrocolloids are highly absorbent gels that are oxygen and water vapor permeable and are often placed on polyurethane films. Depending on their structure they can be very elastic. They are easily cut and can be made as adhesive or nonadhesive. They tend to act as a bacterial barrier and can stay in place for up to 72 hours. These dressings are primarily used for the treatment of venous ulcers, pressure ulcers, first- and second-degree burns, and diabetic/neuropathic ulcers. There are some caveats. Moderately exuding wounds can overwhelm a hydrocolloid dressing in under a day. Another concern in diabetic foot wounds is that hydrocolloids may potentiate anaerobic bacterial growth and, therefore, not recommended for a wound that may harbor anaerobes. Finally, the material that is left on a wound after removing a hydrocolloid dressing has an unpleasant sweet odor that is often mistaken for infection of the wound. However, on balance and for various situations, these dressings are very useful. Commercially available products among many in this category include Replicare, Comfeel, Duoderm, Restore, Nu-Derm, and Curaderm.

FOAM DRESSINGS

Foam dressings are highly absorbent, nonstick dressings made from hydrophilic polyurethane foam. Many of these dressings are waterproof and therefore aid in the prevention of bacterial contamination. The benefit of these high-absorbency dressings is that they can maintain a moist wound environment but not have to be changed frequently. Foam dressings, in general, wick moisture away from the wound, reducing maceration while maintaining a moist wound environment. These dressings come in many forms, are malleable and, thus, can be used in areas that are difficult to dress. These dressings can be left in place for up to 7 days, and they do not leave behind a residual when they are removed. The nonadherent version is very useful in patients with painful wounds such as arterial leg ulcers. In addition, these hydrocellular foams are very efficacious under compression stockings and bandages. One has to be careful as they can produce drying if the wound does not create enough exudate. The best uses for these dressings include heavily exuding wounds, deep cavity wounds, dry heel gangrene, and venous leg ulcers under compression. Commercially available products in this category include, but are not limited to, Allevyn, Biatin, Tielle, Lyofoam, and Curafoam.

ALGINATES

Alginates are frequently used because of their very high absorbency; they are often used in conjunction with numerous other products to control exudates. Alginate is made of soft, nonwoven fibers derived from brown seaweed. Depending on the structure of the product, it can absorb up to 25 times its weight in fluid. As it absorbs this fluid it becomes a gel, and although the various brands differ in their absorbency, the amount of fluid absorbed is directly related to the amount of material applied to the wound. The more absorbent the brand, the more gel-like it becomes over time. Therefore, the more absorbent brands need to be irrigated off, whereas the less absorbent brands can be removed in one piece. The gel itself acts as a vapor-permeable moist wound dressing. In addition, the product has hemostatic properties. The product comes in the form of wound pads or ropes; the latter is very useful in packing deep cavities. There are few drawbacks to alginates. They can dry the wound bed when there is not sufficient exudate. It is necessary to warn patients of the characteristic tan mucous appearance of the dressing. These dressings are excellent for groin wounds that produce a high amount of exudate, or a deep cavitary wound that requires moisture control. The commercially available products in this category include Algisite, Seasorb, Nu-Derm Alginate, Curasorb, Sorbsan, Aquacel, and Hydrofiber.

CHEMICAL DEBRIDEMENT

Chemical debridement refers to the application of topical agents that chemically digest nonvital extracellular proteins that often accumulate in senescent wounds. There are a variety of these agents. Some have proteolytic action, and this is the most studied group. Others denature proteins, and some do both.[18-22] The main components comprising necrotic tissue that develops in chronic and pressure wounds can vary but include keratin, collagen, elastin, proteoglycans and fat.[23] Because of this diversity, it is likely that a group of chemical agents will have the greatest overall efficacy in debriding wounds.

Collagenase

Collagenase is the most studied chemical debrider in the clinical setting. The most common of the collagenases is derived from the fermentation of *Clostridium histolyticum*. Collagen in healthy tissue is not attacked by this agent; collagenase is most effective in wounds with a pH of 6 to 8. Collagenase is deactivated by heavy metals such as silver, which is occasionally used as an antibacterial. When collagenase is applied to the wound, there can be transient local erythema. The collagenase itself should be applied directly to the wound daily and removed by pulse irrigation or washing the wound with a gauze pad. If there is eschar present, it must be crosshatched to allow for penetration of the agent. Collagenase can also be difficult to apply to moist wounds since it is hydrophobic. In studies comparing collagenase with placebo, excellent results have been obtained. On the other hand, collagenase has had mixed results when compared with other wound agents. There are 3 pressure ulcer and 2 chronic wound studies using collagenase that report improved removal of devitalized tissue when compared with placebo.[24-28] However, in a comparative study of collagenase versus DNase and streptokinase in patients with leg ulcers, no statistically significant differences in debridement or healing were observed.[28] Collagenase has also had mixed results when compared with autolytic debridement, and in some cases, autolysis has been found to be superior.[29] Collagenase is available as Santyl Collagenase ointment.

Papain/Urea

The other major chemical debriding agent is papain/urea, which is a combination of a proteolytic enzyme (papain) and a chemical agent (urea) that serves to denature nonviable protein. Papain from papaya is a digestant of nonviable protein and is active over a pH of 3 to 12; however, it requires the stimulator urea to function. The agent may burn when applied. It should be applied directly to the wound, can be washed or irrigated off once or twice a day, and if there is an eschar in the wound, it will need to be crosshatched. In general, papain/urea is easy to apply because it is hydrophilic. In an experimental animal model, papain/urea has been shown to be more efficacious for debridement and wound healing than collagenase or the fibrinolysin-DNase combination.[30] The findings of clinical trials of papain/urea have varied but are usually positive; however, in general, these trials have not been comparative or controlled. The most recent controlled prospective trial assessed 11 patients with chronic pressure ulcers treated with papain/urea versus 10 patients treated with collagenase.[23] In this study, papain/urea was 3 times more effective in reducing the amount of nonviable tissue than the collagenase. However, there were no significant differences in the rate of wound closure or bacterial burden. This product is commercially available as Accuzyme or Gladase.

The one other common agent in this category is a papain/urea-chlorophyllin copper complex. This agent is bright green, application can be from once a day to every 72 hours, and it can be applied under pressure dressings. It is a good adjunct to the standard papain/urea products because it tends to burn less than the standard papain/urea combinations. However, there is little outcomes literature to support its use over other agents. This agent is currently available as Panafil.

BACTERIAL BURDEN

The bacterial burden of a chronic wound is an important determinant of its ability to heal. The mere presence of bacteria in a chronic wound does not indicate infection or that the bacteria are impairing wound healing, or that the wound needs to be treated with antibiotics.[31,32] The presence of microorganisms in the wound in low levels may actually facilitate healing and enhance autolytic debridement.[33,34] Bacteria in a wound bed under a moist wound care dressing produce proteolytic enzymes such as hyaluronidase, which not only act as debriders but stimulate neutrophils to release proteases.[35] The organisms that are acquired by chronic wounds can be either indigenous flora or external from the environment. The 4 categories of bacterial involvement of a wound include wound contamination, wound colonization, critical colonization, and wound infection.

Wound contamination is defined as the presence of nonreplicating microorganisms in the wound. In contrast, wound colonization is the presence of replicating microorganisms that are adherent to the wound but do not cause injury to the host. These are most often the skin flora such as *Staphylococcus epidermidis* and *Corynebacterium*.[36] Critical colonization occurs when bacteria cause a delay in wound healing.[37,38] Bacteria not only release useful proteolytic enzymes, but they also can release MMPs and other inflammatory mediators that can impair the healing process. In this setting, epithelializaion will fail to occur, and there may be an increased serous exudate, as well as the development of bright red exuberant granulation tissue. This latter response is secondary to bacteria's ability to stimulate angiogenesis. This granulation tissue, however, has deficient matrix that is overly friable and prone to bleeding. In this setting, dressing changes are often accompanied by bleeding and an unpleasant odor. In addition, wounds affected by bacteria may exhibit new areas of wound breakdown or necrosis.[39]

The diagnosis of wound infection is difficult. However, it should be considered when any wound fails to heal or there is progressive deterioration. Signs and symptoms of deep tissue infections include increased pain or the presence of pain in a neuropathic wound, increased size, surrounding warmth and erythema, and the presence of exposed bone. If there is uncertainty, a tissue biopsy should be performed. The 2 methods used are the quantitative biopsy and curettage of tissue from the base of a debrided ulcer. In both cases, the wound is cleaned with saline and debrided with gauze. In the quantitative biopsy, 1 mm^3 of tissue is excised from the area in question; sometimes up to 4 areas from a wound are chosen, depending on the size. This method evaluates the presence of microorganisms within the tissue versus on the surface. Because quantitative biopsy is time-consuming and invasive, it is often reserved for wounds that have not responded to all other methods of treatment and in preparation for skin grafts. The curettage method involves scraping of the wound bed with the edge of a ten blade; the matrix is then swabbed off the blade and plated. This will give the clinician information about the type of flora present but not the quantity. In some microbiology laboratories, bacterial growth can be reported semi-quantitatively as 1 to 4+, with 4+ growth correlating well with wounds that have greater than 10^5 colony-forming units (CFU) of bacteria per gram of tissue. This has been shown to be a threshold representing active infection. In numerous studies, the quantitative bacterial burden has been noted to be a key element in the speed and completeness of wound healing. Browne et al[38] demonstrated that in patients with diabetic nonhealing ulcers treated with an engineered skin substitute, the wound healing rate for those with no growth on quantitative culture was 0.20 cm/wk; for those with 10^5 to 10^6 CFU per gram of tissue, the healing rate was 0.15 cm/wk; and for those with greater than 10^6 CFU per gram of tissue, the healing rate was 0.055 cm/wk.[40]

Many factors other than the quantity of bacteria produce wound infection versus critical colonization. They include the host's ability to resist infection, which is affected by many factors such as the presence of diabetes, cancer, malnutrition, impaired hepatic function, and the use of systemic steroids. The virulence of the bacteria can be as much of a factor as the quantity of the bacteria present. The microbial environment of the chronic wound changes over time. In the early stages, normal skin flora predominate including *Staphylococcus aureus* and β-hemolytic streptococci. After 4 weeks, the chronic wound becomes colonized with facultative anaerobic gram-negative rods such as *Proteus, Escherichia coli*, and *Klebsiella*. As the deeper tissues become involved, anaerobic organisms become an inhabitant of chronic wounds.[41] Wounds of several months duration often have 4 to 5 different pathogens present, and these may include *Pseudomonas, Acinetobacter*, and *Stenotrophomonas* species. Interestingly, these seldom cause soft tissue invasion unless the host is highly compromised.[42] Certain organisms require treatment no matter their density. These include β-hemolytic streptococci, mycobacteria, *Bacillus anthracis, Yersinia pestis, Corynebacterium diphtheriae, Erysipelothrix, Leptospira, Treponema, Brucella*, herpesvirus, *Histoplasma, Blastomyces, Coccidioides,* and parasitic organisms such as leishmaniasis.[42]

When to use antimicrobial therapy for wounds is often controversial. Contaminated and colonized wounds do not need treatment. Obviously, enhancing the host's ability to fight infection is a paramount step and includes such strategies as revascularization, glucose control, and control of edema. In addition, the removal of foreign bodies and devascularized and necrotic tissue (soft tissue, bone, fascia, muscle, and ligament) is mandatory when attempting to improve local host defenses.[43] The removal of foreign material greatly increases the concentration of microorganisms necessary to produce an infection.[44] Once appropriate debridement has been accomplished, the next steps that will decrease the bacterial burden include wound disinfection, topical antimicrobial therapy, and systemic antimicrobial therapy.

WOUND CLEANING

Physiologic saline applied to the wound bed at pressures between 8 and 15 psi can remove microbes without disturbing healthy tissue. The addition of antibiotics or disinfecting agents to these solutions is not necessary. In general, the use of pulsatile lavage has been shown experimentally to reduce the quantitative bacterial count by a factor of 10^2.[45]

WOUND DISINFECTION

Most agents available for wound disinfection have been shown to be toxic to wound fibroblasts. This toxicity varies between agents and can be modified greatly by changes in concentration.[46-49] The most commonly used disinfectants include povidone-iodine, chlorhexidine, alcohol, acetic acid, hydrogen peroxide, and sodium hypochlorite (Dakin's solution). Dilute solutions of the following have been shown to aid in the healing of wounds during the most active phase of infection: sodium hypochlorite at 0.005% concentration, acetic acid at 0.0025% concentration, and povidone-iodine at 0.09% concentration. At these concentrations, the solutions can all be bactericidal while allowing fibroblast growth. In a wound that is compromised by the presence of hematoma, dilute hydrogen peroxide is anecdotally useful as well. One novel agent that allows for the slow decontamination of a wound is cadexomer iodine. The modified starch matrix absorbs wound exudate into its cadexomer polymer-gel. As the gel expands, 9% elemental iodine is slowly released. At 72 hours, a color change from brown to gray demonstrates that all the active iodine has been released.[50]

TOPICAL ANTIMICROBIAL THERAPY

Topical antimicrobials are the agents that can be used in critically colonized wounds, or in conjunction with systemic antibiotics in infected wounds. The general precept governing the use of topical antimicrobials is that they should have a low potential for sensitization, not be used systemically, and have low tissue toxicity.[51] Many topical agents are available, including silver sulfadiazine, neomycin, polymyxin B, gentamicin, gentamicin beads, mupirocin, 5% mafenide acetate, and dressings that use nanocrystalline silver technology. To date, very few data support the use of any of these agents. A detailed description of these agents and the studies evaluating their utility are beyond the scope of this chapter.

SYSTEMIC ANTIMICROBIAL THERAPY

Systemic antimicrobial therapy is reserved for the infected wound, and can be used in conjunction with topical therapy. In the compromised chronic wound, tissue levels of antibiotic will often be nontherapeutic despite achieving adequate systemic levels; therefore, a combination of the 2 modalities might be useful. Appropriate antibiotics are chosen based on culture data and host factors, including allergies. In general, the choice between intravenous and oral therapy is determined by the severity and systemic characteristics of the infection, the organisms involved, and the presence or absence of bone or joint involvement. Most algorithms for soft tissue infections define courses of 2 weeks on average, with some chronic infections requiring up to 12 weeks of therapy.[32]

ADVANCED WOUND HEALING STRATEGIES

Most of the agents and techniques that we have discussed to this point have been methods that modify the wound environment. In sum, optimal preparation of the wound bed requires complete debridement of devitalized tissue, moisture, and control of bacterial levels. Host factors need to be assessed and treated. Other relevant factors that require maximization include nutrition, pressure, oxygen delivery, and edema. In this setting, most wounds will heal. However, if all of these issues have been addressed and the wound still fails to heal, there are numerous products and devices that reach beyond those that simply prepare the wound bed. Products that fall in this category include biomaterial wound modifiers, engineered skin substitutes, topical growth factors, and other adjunctive therapies.

BIOMATERIAL WOUND MODIFIERS

Biomaterials for the treatment of wounds are biologic materials that do not produce an immune-mediated response but prevent infection and enhance wound healing. The 2 agents that deserve mention in this category are small intestinal submucosa (SIS) and oxidized regenerated cellulose (ORC)/collagen.

SIS

SIS is sterilized to eliminate cell-borne pathogens and has a long shelf-life. SIS is extracellular matrix derived from the terminal small intestine of pigs. Present are primarily proteins with small amounts of carbohydrate and lipids, collagen (types I, III, VI), glycosaminoglycans, proteoglycans, and glycoproteins. SIS is thought to aid in wound healing by providing a 3-dimensional structure that acts as a scaffold for host tissue remodeling. The preparations that are minimally antigenic are gradually colonized by host tissue cells, blood vessels, and additional extracellular matrix.[52,53] Preclinical studies have demonstrated enhanced healing when SIS is used as a matrix to replace full-thickness defects in the skin of rats.[54] This structure formed a stratified squamous epithelium after only 10 days. The clinical application of SIS is most interesting. SIS has been used to treat first- and second-degree burns, trauma, and surgical wounds. Brown-Etris et al[55] compared SIS with the standard of care for the treatment of full-thickness pressure ulcers, with the outcome measures being complete healing and pain. In both categories, SIS was superior to the standard of care. Others have found similar results.[56] SIS dressings are applied with clean technique. The dressing is cut slightly larger than the wound and requires rehydration with physiologic saline. A moist environment is necessary, and the wound should be inspected at least weekly. It is not uncommon to observe a caramel-colored gel on the wound bed. This is a normal reaction to the combination of SIS and the host's body fluid. This gel should be gently irrigated and not forcibly removed, as budding epithelial cells may be disturbed. SIS is available as Oasis from Healthpoint.

ORC/Collagen

ORC/collagen was developed as a biopolymer with performance properties designed to promote healing of chronic wounds. These properties include the ability to attract cells to the wound site; promotion of cell proliferation, migration, and matrix protein production; normalization of the proteolytic imbalance of the chronic wound; neutralization of factors that inhibit growth; the ability to bind growth factors; and the ability to bioresorb.[57,58] In a diabetic mouse model, ORC/collagen produced an accelerated healing response.[59] This agent has also been shown to bind significantly more MMPs for longer than either control or gauze but, as of yet, no clinical trials have assessed this product. A randomized trial will be necessary to determine its true potential. The matrix is applied after being hydrated with saline, applied directly to the wound bed, and then covered with a secondary dressing to maintain a moist wound healing environment. It can be reapplied at 1- to 3-day intervals depending on the level of exudate. This product is available as Promogran from Johnson and Johnson.

TOPICAL GROWTH FACTORS

The application of topical growth factors to chronic wounds is based on the concept that either there is a deficiency in the quantity of growth factors present in chronic wounds, or that enhancement of a preexisting growth factor will improve wound healing. Growth factors, however, work in concert, and differing growth factors are necessary at the various phases of wound healing. The topical growth factors that have been evaluated include basic fibroblast growth factor (bFGF; stimulates endothelial cell proliferation and migration), transforming growth factor-β (TGF-β; stimulates fibroblasts and keratinocytes and the production of collagen), epidermal growth factor (EGF; supports the growth of keratinocytes and assists in the migration of keratinocytes, fibroblasts, and endothelial cells), keratinocyte growth factor-2 (KGF-2; stimulates the growth of normal epithelial keratinocytes), platelet-derived growth factor (PDGF; chemotactic for polymorphonuclear neutrophils and macrophages), and vascular endothelial growth factor (VEGF; stimulates epithelial proliferation and granulation).

PDGF is available in a commercial formulation that contains recombinant human PDGF (rhPDGF) in an aqueous-based sodium carboxymethylcellulose gel. The efficacy of this agent has been supported by numerous clinical trials.[60] The gel is applied directly to granulating wounds under a moist dressing, and should be wiped off after 12 hours and recovered with a moist dressing until the next morning's application. This product is available by prescription as Regranex gel. Another novel way to introduce PDGF is in conjunction with ORC/collagen as a once-a-day dressing. ORC/collagen will release PDGF as it dissolves. New clinical trials are also underway to assess the efficacy of topical VEGF in the treatment of noninfected diabetic foot wounds. Moreover, a recent clinical trial that assessed the treatment of chronic venous stasis ulcers with KGF-2 appears to have demonstrated little or no efficacy of this agent for treating wounds. Nevertheless, the assessment of growth factors in the treatment of wounds will actively continue via both animal and clinical studies for some time to come.

Topical application of gene therapy to deliver growth factors to chronic wounds is another approach being used in the treatment of chronic wounds. Animal studies involving ischemic wound models suggest that a single application of adenoviral vectors expressing PDGF accelerates healing at the same rate as the daily application of PDGF. Clinical trials are underway. This mode of therapy may offer many benefits over daily topical therapy, including lower cost and better patient compliance.[42]

ENGINEERED SKIN SUBSTITUTES

Skin grafts and rotational flaps leave large defects behind, and in the compromised host may simply result in another wound problem. For years, attempts have been made to culture and grow keratinocytes to facilitate the closure of acute and chronic wounds without the creation of another wound. Bioengineered skin substitutes replace the patient's own skin by providing a matrix with living cells that stimulates the patient's own epithelial cells. Skin substitutes do not work like an allograft in that they require 5 to 8 weekly applications. Alternatively, no anesthesia or suturing is required.

One commercially available skin substitute is composed of human dermal fibroblasts obtained from neonatal foreskin. These cells are seeded onto a bioabsorbable polyglactin mesh that serves as a scaffolding.[61] Fibroblasts proliferate within the scaffolding, secreting human collagens, glycosaminoglycans, and other dermal proteins. A sheet of dermal tissue containing metabolically active cells and a human dermal matrix is eventually formed.[62] Once complete, this engineered graft is cryopreserved and frozen at −70°C until implantation. A controlled, prospective, randomized, blinded, multicenter trial using bioengineered skin was performed in 281 patients with full-thickness diabetic neuropathic ulcers (>1 cm^2).[63] The median time to healing was 13 weeks for patients receiving the skin substitute versus 28 weeks for controls. In addition, the median time to recurrence was 12 weeks in the skin substitute group and 7 weeks in the control group, with similar wound infection rates of 20% in both groups. This product is currently marketed as Dermagraft from Smith and Nephew.

Another skin substitute is an allogenic bilayered tissue consisting of a layer of viable keratinocytes and a dermal layer of viable fibroblasts embedded in a type I collagen matrix. It also appears to have good clinical efficacy in venous leg ulcers and in neuropathic diabetic foot ulcers.[64] This product does not require thawing, has little preparation time, and is easy to apply. However, it is also the most costly of the commercially available skin substitutes. It is marketed as Apligraf and is distributed by Novartis. It is the only skin substitute approved for venous stasis ulcers, although other products are probably equally efficacious. The results of a recent clinical trial of the treatment of venous stasis ulcers with a bilayered cellular matrix consisting of a collagen sponge seeded with allogenic keratinocytes and fibroblasts are being analyzed. However, preservation of keratinocyte and fibroblast viability, ease of application, and cost are all problems that remain to be dealt with before these products will become widely applied. At present, they are best reserved for those patients in whom all other forms of therapy short of skin grafting have failed.

ADJUNCTIVE THERAPIES
Negative Pressure Wound Therapy

Negative pressure wound therapy (NPWT) involves the placement of an open-cell foam dressing into the wound cavity and applying controlled subatmospheric pressure. The technique removes chronic edema, increases local blood flow, and enhances formation of granulation tissue.[65,66] Single-center studies have demonstrated that NPWT can enhance granulation tissue and decrease the depth of wounds.[67] Currently, several industry-sponsored clinical trials evaluating NPWT for the treatment of venous stasis, diabetic foot and trunk pressure ulcers, as well as sternal wounds, are underway. This product is available from KCI as the V.A.C.

Electrical Stimulation and Ultrasound

Electrical stimulation has been shown to activate fibroblasts and stimulate the migration of other key cells.[68] There are 25 reports in the literature in which electrical stimulation has been used in the treatment of chronic wounds. Ten of these studies are randomized, and all demonstrate benefit of this electrical stimulation in wound healing. In vitro studies have shown that therapeutic ultrasound can lead to the release of chemoattractants and mitogenic factors, with resulting enhancement of fibroblast proliferation and collagen synthesis. There are 12 randomized, controlled trials in which ultrasound has been used to treat chronic wounds, and 8 of the trials have been positive.[42]

Other adjunctive therapies include electromagnetic fields, pneumatic compression, therapeutic heat, hydrotherapy, and laser. However, there are not sufficient clinical data available with any of these techniques to justify their current clinical use.

WOUND TREATMENT ALGORITHMS

The foregoing is a relatively comprehensive review of the field of wound healing. However, the question of how and when to apply these numerous techniques remains. In practice, one should first assess the patient for systemic factors that might affect wound healing. Laboratory tests might include hemoglobin (maintain >10 g/dL), albumin (prealbumin, transferrin), a chemistry panel, and HbA_{1c}. A 3-day diary is recorded assessing intake of proteins, calories, and carbohydrates. Pain needs to be managed, and surrounding skin care issues are addressed. The cleanliness of the wound is then evaluated. If there is a clinical suspicion of infection, the wound is cultured. Necrotic tissue is sharply debrided, and if necessary, this should be accomplished in the operating room with pulse irrigation. The next step is the assessment of etiology. Is the wound arterial, neuropathic, from venous stasis, or from a combination of these etiologies? The fundamental underlying problem should then be addressed, such as control of edema or revascularization. The appearance of the wound should allow its placement in a descriptive group. For example, the wound is clean with a granular base or a crater; there is necrotic/nonviable tissue; the wound has an exudate; there is a sinus; or the wound is infected. The wound with a clean granular base is most often treated with a hydrogel, as the primary objective is to protect the wound and keep it moist. Other options for this type of wound include hydrocolloid dressings. The wound with a crater is often treated with a hydrogel or NPWT, as the primary objective is to fill in the crater. Wounds with necrotic/nonviable tissue are primarily treated with chemical debriders, or hydrocolloids allowing for autolytic debridement, since debriding and cleansing of the wound are the primary goals. Other options for these wounds include pulse irrigation and NPWT. Wounds with exudate are best treated with alginates, foams, or NPWT, to absorb and contain the drainage. For the wound with a sinus, tunnel, or that is undermined, calcium alginate rope, NPWT, or a gauze impregnated with a hydrogel are the best options. Wounds with infection are best treated with topical antibiotics, or if heavily contaminated they can be treated with a wound disinfectant for a limited time, followed by a topical antimicrobial.

CONCLUSION

The effective treatment of chronic wounds is based on having a thorough understanding of the differences between chronic and acute wounds. Once these differences are understood, evaluation of the host and improvement of underlying predisposing conditions are mandatory—for example, by revascularization of an ischemic limb, controlling venous reflux, or off-loading a neuropathic ulcer. Preparing the wound bed is the next step and includes removal of devitalized tissue, maintenance of a moist wound environment, and controlling the bacterial burden. Once these goals have been achieved, most wounds will heal without further intervention. However, for those that do not, other modalities include growth factors or biomaterials, and for the most recalcitrant wounds, bioengineered skin substitutes are available.

It is with a large armamentarium of treatments that we tackle the problem of complex chronic wounds. Unfortunately, there are few prospective, randomized data to guide our approach. It can still be rightly called the "art of wound healing."

REFERENCES

1. Lazarus GS, Cooper DM, Knighton DR, et al: Definitions and guidelines for assessment of wounds and evaluation of healing. *Arch Dermatol* 130:489-493, 1994.
2. Seiler WO, Staehlin HB, Zolliker R, et al: Impaired migration of epidermal cells from decubitus ulcers in cell cultures: A cause of protracted wound healing? *Am J Clin Pathol* 92:430-434, 1989.
3. Himmel HN: Wound healing: Focus on the chronic wound. *Wounds* 7:70A-77A, 1995.
4. Winter GD: Formation of the scab and rate of epithelialisation of superficial wounds in the skin of the young domestic pig. *Nature* 193:293-294, 1962.
5. Falanga V: Classifications of wound preparation and stimulation of chronic wounds. *Wound Repair Regen* 8:347-352, 2000.
6. Paloahti M, Lauharanta L, Stephens RW, et al: Proteolytic activity in leg ulcer exudates. *Exp Dermatol* 2:29-37, 1993.
7. Kirsner RS, Katz MH, Eaglstein WH, et al: The biology of wound fluid. *Wounds* 3:122-128, 1993.
8. Bucalo B, Eaglstein WH, Falanga V: Inhibition of cell proliferation by chronic wound fluid. *Wound Repair Regen* 1:181-186, 1993.
9. Falanga V: Wound bed preparation and the role of enzymes: A case for multiple actions of therapeutic agents. *Wounds* 14:47-57, 2002.
10. Sibbald RG, Williamson D, Orsted HL, et al: Preparing the wound bed: Debridement, bacterial balance, and moisture balance. *Ostomy Wound Manage* 46:14-35, 2000.
11. Szycher M, Lee SJ: Wound dressings: A systematic approach to wound healing. *J Biomater Appl* 7:142-213, 1992.
12. Alvarez O, Rozint J, Meehan M: Principles of moist wound healing: Indications for chronic, in Krasner D (ed): *Chronic Wound Care: A Clinical Source Book for Healthcare Professionals.* King of Prussia, Pa, Health Management Publications, 1990, pp 266-281.
13. Haimowitz JE, Margolis DJ: Moist wound healing, in Krasner D, Kane D (eds): *Chronic Wound Care: A Clinical Source Book for Healthcare Professionals*, ed 2. Wayne, Pa, Health Management Publications, 1997, pp 49-56.

14. Hinman CD, Maibach H: Effect of air exposure and occlusion on experimental human skin wounds. *Nature* 200:377-379, 1963.

15. Winter GD: Healing of skin wounds and the influence of dressings on the repair process, in Harkiss (ed): *Surgical Dressings and Wound Healing*. Bradford, England, Bradford University Press, 1971, pp 46-60.

16. Hutchinson JJ: Prevalence of wound infection under occlusive dressings: A collective survey of reported research. *J Hosp Infect* 17:83-94, 1991.

17. Field CK, Kerstein MD: Overview of wound healing in a moist environment. *Am J Surg* 167:2S-6S, 1994.

18. Westerhof W: Future prospects of proteolytic enzymes and wound healing, in Westerhof W, Vanscheidt W (eds): *Proteolytic Enzymes and Wound Healing*. New York, Springer-Verlag, 1994, pp 99-102.

19. Levenson SM, Gruber DK, Gruber C, et al: Chemical debridement of burns: Mercaptans. *J Trauma* 21:632-644, 1981.

20. Burke JF, Golden T: A clinical evaluation of enzymatic debridement with papain/urea-chlorophillin ointment. *Am J Surg* 95:828-842, 1958.

21. Levenson SM: Debriding agents. *J Trauma* 19:928S-930S, 1979.

22. Falabella A: Debridement of wounds. *Wounds* 10:1C-9C, 1998.

23. Alvarez OM, Fernandez-Obregon A, Rogers RS, et al: Chemical debridement of pressure ulcers: A prospective, randomized, comparative trial of collagenase and papain/urea formulations. *Wounds* 12:15-25, 2000.

24. Rao DB, Sane PG, Georgiev EL: Collagenase in the treatment of dermal and decubitus ulcers. *J Am Geriatr Soc* 23:22-30, 1975.

25. Varma AO, Bugatch E: Debridement of dermal ulcers with collagenase. *Surg Gynecol Obstet* 136:281-282, 1973.

26. Boxer AM, Gottesman N, Bersnstein H, et al: Debridement of dermal ulcers and decubiti with collagenase. *Geriatrics* 24:75-86, 1969.

27. Lee LK, Ambrus JL: Collagenase therapy for decubitus ulcers. *Geriatrics* 30:91-98, 1975.

28. Westerhof W, Jansen FC, deWit FS: Controlled double blind trail of fibrinolysin-deoxyribonuclease (Elase) solution in patients with chronic leg ulcers who are treated before autologous skin grafting. *J Am Acad Dermatol* 17:32-38, 1987.

29. Brown-Etris M, Punthello M, Shields D, et al: A comparison clinical study to evaluate the efficacy of 80% hypertonic wound gel dressing vs. collagenase ointment for the debridement of non-viable tissue in dermal ulcers. Presented at the 11th Annual Symposium on Advanced Wound Care and Medical Research Forum on Wound Repair, Miami, Fla, April 18-22, 1998.

30. Hebda PA, Flynn KJ, Dohar JE: Evaluation of efficacy of enzymatic debriding agents for the removal of necrotic tissue and promotion of healing in porcine skin wounds. *Wounds* 10:83-96, 1998.

31. Kerstein MD: The scientific basis of healing. *Adv Wound Care* 10:30-36, 1997.

32. Dow G, Browne A, Sibbald RG: Infection in chronic wounds: Controversies in diagnosis and treatment. *Ostomy Wound Manage* 45:23-40, 1999.

33. DeHaan BB, Ellis H, Wilkes M: The role of infection in wound healing. *Surg Gynecol Obstet* 138:693-700, 1974.

34. Pollack SV: The wound healing process. *Clin Dermatol* 29:83-92, 1984.

35. Stone LL: Bacterial debridement of the burn eschar: The in vivo activity of selected organisms. *J Surg Res* 29:83-92, 1980.

36. Rodeheaver G, Smith S, Thacker J, et al: Mechanical cleansing of contaminated wounds with a surfactant. *Am J Surg* 129:241-245, 1975.

37. Sibbald RG, Browne AC, Coutts P, et al: Screening evaluation of an ionized nanocrystalline silver dressing in chronic wound care. *Ostomy Wound Manage* 47:38-43, 2001.

38. Browne AC, Vearncombe M, Sibbald AG: High bacterial load in asymptomatic diabetic patients with neuropathic ulcers retards wound healing after application of Dermagraft. *Ostomy Wound Manage* 47:44-49, 2001.

39. Cutting KF, Harding KGH: Criteria for identifying wound infection. *J Wound Care* 3:198-201, 1994.

40. Robson MC, Krizek TJ: Predicting skin graft survival. *J Trauma* 13:213-217, 1973.

41. Bowler PG, Duerden BI, Armstrong DG: Wound microbiology and associated approaches to wound management. *Clin Microbiol Rev* 14:244-269, 2001.

42. Schultz GS, Sibbald RG, Falanga V, et al: Wound bed preparation: A systematic approach to wound management. *Wound Repair Regen* 11:1-28, 2003.

43. Elek S: Experimental staphylococcal infections in the skin of man. *Ann N Y Acad Sci* 65:85-90, 1956.

44. Elek SD: The virulence of staph pyogenes for man: A study of wound infection. *Br J Exp Pathol* 38:573-586, 1957.

45. Rodeheaver G: Wound cleansing, wound irrigation, wound disinfection, in Krasner D, Kane D (eds): *Chronic Wound Care: A Clinical Source Book for Healthcare Professional*, ed 2. Wayne, Pa, Health Management Publications, 1997, pp 97-109.

46. Eaglestein WH, Falanga V: Chronic wounds. *Surg Clin North Am* 77:689-700, 1997.

47. Falanga V: Iodine containing pharmaceuticals: A reappraisal, in *Proceedings of the 6th European Conference on the Advances in Wound Management*, Amsterdam, Oct 1-4, 1996, pp 191-194.

48. Viljanto J: Disinfection of surgical wounds without inhibition of normal wound healing. *Arch Surg* 115:253-256, 1980.

49. Gruber RP, Vistnes L, Pardue R: The effect of the commonly used antiseptics on wound healing. *Plast Reconstr Surg* 55:472-476, 1975.

50. Moberg S, Hoffman L, Grennert M, et al: A randomized trial of cadexomer iodine in decubitus ulcers. *J Am Geriatr Soc* 31:462-465, 1983.

51. Boyce ST, Holder IA: Selection of topical antimicrobial agents for cultured skin for burns: Combined assessment of cellular cytotoxicity and antimicrobial activity. *Plast Reconstr Surg* 92:493-500, 1993.

52. Voytik-Harbin SL, Brightman AO, Kraine M, et al: Identification of extractable growth factors from small intestinal submucosa. *J Cell Biochem* 67:478-491, 1997.

53. Hodde JP, Badylak SF, Brightman AO, et al: Glycosaminoglycan content of small intestinal submucosa: A bioscaffold for tissue replacement. *Tissue Eng* 2:209-217, 1996.

54. Prevel CD, Eppley BL, Summerlin DJ, et al: Small intestinal submucosa: Utilization as a wound dressing in full thickness rodent wounds. *Ann Plast Surg* 35:381-388, 1995.

55. Brown-Etris M, Punchello M, Milne C, et al: Clinical update: Evaluation of small intestinal submucosa (SIS) in the treatment of full thickness pressure ulcers. Presented at the Wound Healing Society Educational Symposium and Exhibition, Baltimore, Md, May 2002.

56. Niezgoda JA, Frykberg RG, Parmater M, et al: Evaluation of Oasis wound dressing for treating full thickness diabetic ulcers. Presented at the European Tissue Repair Society Annual Meeting, Cardiff, Wales, September 2001.

57. Cullen B, Watt PW, Lundquist C, et al: The role of oxidized regenerated cellulose/collagen in chronic wound repair and its potential mechanism of action. *Int J Biochem Cell Biol* 34:1544-1556, 2002.

58. Cullen B, Clark R, McCulloch E, et al: The effect of PROMOGRAN, a novel biomaterial, on protease activities present in wound fluid collected from decubitus ulcers. *Wound Repair Regen* 9:407, 2001.

59. Hart J, Silcock D, Gunnigle S, et al: The role of oxidized regenerated cellulose/collagen in wound repair: Effects in vitro on fibroblast biology and in vivo in a model of compromised healing. *Int J Biochem Cell Biol* 34:1557-1570, 2002.

60. Steed DL: Clinical evaluation of recombinant human platelet derived growth factor for the treatment of lower extremity diabetic ulcers. Diabetic ulcer study group. *J Vasc Surg* 21:71-81, 1995.

61. Cooper ML, Hansborough JF, Spievogel RL, et al: In vivo optimization of a living dermis substitute employing cultured human fibroblasts on a biodegradable polyglycolic acid or polyglactin mesh. *Biomaterials* 12:243-248, 1991.

62. Landeen LK, Ziegler FC, Halberstadt C, et al: Characterization of a human dermal replacement. *Wounds* 4:167-175, 1992.

63. Pollak RA, Edington H, Jensen JL, et al: A human dermal replacement for the treatment of diabetic foot ulcers. *Wounds* 9:175-183, 1997.

64. Falanga V: Apligraf treatment of venous ulcers and other chronic wounds. *J Dermatol* 25:812-817, 1998.

65. Argenta LC, Morykwas MJ: Vacuum-assisted closure: A new method for wound control and treatment: Clinical experience. *Ann Plast Surg* 348:563-576, 1997.

66. Morykwas MJ, Argenta LC, Shelton-Brown EI, et al: Vacuum-assisted closure: A new method for wound control and treatment: Animal studies and basic foundation. *Ann Plast Surg* 38:553-562, 1997.
67. Joseph E, Hamori CA, Bergamn S, et al: A prospective randomized trial of vacuum-assisted closure versus standard therapy of chronic non-healing wounds. *Wounds* 12:60-67, 2000.
68. Thawer HA, Houghton PE: Effects of electrical stimulation on the histological properties of wounds in diabetic mice. *Wound Repair Regen* 9:107-115, 2001.

Index

Page numbers followed by italic *f* or *t* indicate figures or tables, respectively.

Information and insights you won't find anywhere else—straight from the experts!

YES! Please start my subscription to the *Advances* checked below with the current volume according to the terms described below.* I understand that I will have 30 days to examine each annual edition.

Please Print:

Name _____

Address _____

City _____ State _____ ZIP _____

Method of Payment

❑ Check (payable to **Elsevier**; add the applicable sales tax for your area)

❑ VISA ❑ MasterCard ❑ AmEx ❑ Bill me

Card number _____ Exp. date _____

Signature _____

❑ **Advances in Anesthesia® (YAAN)**
$111.00 (Avail. December)

❑ **Advances in Dermatology® (YADR)**
$111.00 (Avail. November)

❑ **Advances in Pediatrics® (YAPD)**
$101.00 (Avail. July)

❑ **Advances in Surgery® (YASU)**
$101.00 (Avail. September)

❑ **Advances in Vascular Surgery® (YAVS)**
$101.00 (Avail. October)

Order your *Advances* today! Simply complete and detach this card and drop it in the mail to receive the latest information in your field.

*Your Advances service guarantee:

When you subscribe to an *Advances*, you will receive notice of future annual volumes about two months before publication. To receive the new edition, do nothing—we'll send you the new volume as soon as it is available. (Applicable sales tax is added to each shipment.) If you want to discontinue, the advance notice allows you time to notify us of your decision. If you are not completely satisfied, you have 30 days to return any *Advances*.

VISIT OUR HOME PAGE!
www.us.elsevierhealth.com/periodicals

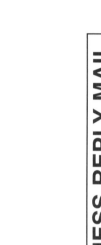

ELSEVIER
MOSBY